CON

Caring for Elderly Parents

zurBurg

Henry Holstege

TRADING PLACES

CRC Publications
Grand Rapids, Michigan

© 1996 by CRC Publications, 2850 Kalamazoo Ave. SE, Grand Rapids, Michigan 49560.

Library of Congress Cataloging-in-Publication Data
Holstege, Henry, 1932-
    Trading Places: caring for elderly parents/Henry Holstege.
        p. cm.—(Issues in Christian Living)
    Includes bibliographical references.
    ISBN 1-56212-171-5
    1. Aging parents — United States. 2. Aging parents — Care—United States. 3. Parents and adult child—United States. 4. Caregivers—United States. 5. Intergenerational relations—United States. 6. Aging parents—Care—Religious aspects—Christianity. I. Title. II. Series.
HQ1063.6.H65   1996
306.874—dc20   96-12780
                                                              CIP

10 9 8 7 6 5 4 3 2 1

INTRODUCTION

"Auntie, you have the same color hair as Grandma's." That observation from a six-year-old was neither news nor comfort to the listener who was too old to blame "premature graying" and too young to claim "senior" discounts. And little did the child know that she had aptly described part of a phenomenon called "the graying of North America."

Demographic trends point toward an "age wave" created by the simultaneous growing number of elderly people, the decrease in the birth rate, and the aging of the baby boomers (Dychtwald and Fowler, 1990 as reported in *Christian Education Journal*, Winter 1995, p. 37). Today older people make up a significant proportion of the population in the United States and Canada. The percentage of Americans who are sixty-five and older has tripled from 4.1 percent in 1900, to 12.5 percent of the American population in 1990. In fact, the fastest growing age category in the United States is those eighty-five and older. Although Canada's aging population has not increased at the same rate as in the United States, the percentage of older persons has more than doubled since the turn of the century from about 5 percent to 11.6 percent in 1991.

Life expectancy at the turn of the century was less than fifty. Today, life expectancy in the United States is approaching seventy-eight for women and seventy-two for men. A million U.S. baby boomers (those born between 1946 and 1964) are expected to celebrate their

100th birthdays. The average life expectancy for Canadians is seventy-eight years.

Indeed, the family album is changing. Because middle-aged adults often have living parents, the phrase "sandwich generation" means more to them than feasting on deli submarines with everything to go! And before long, our family portraits will probably include three or four living generations from the youngest great-grandchild to the oldest great (even great-great) grandparent, often with one or more "middle" generations "sandwiched" in between, feeling the pressures of trying to balance the needs of both young and old.

We, like the observant—and blunt—six-year-old, are probably discovering that gray is "in" and here to stay. Everyone from families, to business and industry, to government has been affected by this age wave. Futurists predict major changes in our North American culture as we redirect our focus from youth to the problems and needs of an aging population. These changes will not come without stress and intergenerational conflict, even on the home front.

Looking around our congregations, most of us can see that the church has not escaped this graying process. However, researchers indicate that "the church has been one of the slowest institutions to respond to the issue of an aging population" even though church membership, especially in rural areas, includes about 10 percent more elderly than the total community ("Older-Adult Ministry: Preparation for the Future," Ronnie Johnson, *Christian Education Journal,* Winter 1995, pp. 37-38). Churches have a dual challenge: responding to the needs of aging members themselves and supporting those families who are caring for elderly parents in varied situations. And certainly there is the ongoing "mission" to develop and nurture in all of us a sense of intergenerational love and appreciation, a demonstration of acceptance and caring.

This book was written to help you and other members of your church family explore some issues surrounding the aging of our society, and to help you deal with the day-to-day reality of this process in your own life and family. The material is designed for small group discussion as well as personal reflection. We hope that each of the six sessions will increase a sense of communion—an intergenerational interdependence—within your church family and also renewed appreciation for blessings that come from sharing our personal needs and concerns with others. We also hope you will find helpful information that will assist you in caring for your own elderly parents, often as you find yourself *Trading Places* with them.

ONE

THE SANDWICH GENERATION

- *Hello, I'm Alice. I'm a forty-eight-year-old wife, mother, and sixth-grade teacher. My husband, a high school teacher, and I have three children ages sixteen, twenty-two, and twenty-five. Jack's parents are in their late seventies, still in good health, although his mother is becoming quite forgetful. My mother recently had a stroke and needs daily transportation for physical therapy. My father has Parkinson's disease and no longer drives. My only brother and his family live nearby. We've decided it's time to call our two sisters who live out of state. I'm so stressed. . . . How are we going to take care of Dad and Mom?*

- *My name is Don. I'm a fifty-year-old attorney. My father, eighty-five, is bedridden, in the latter stages of Alzheimer's. For the past five years, he's been in a nursing home in my hometown—a thousand miles from here. My mother, eighty-two, is very frail and suffering from osteoporosis. My only sister lives in the same town as Dad and Mom. She's been calling often lately, worried about how much longer Mom can live alone and if their money will last. She wants me to come home. But I'm under so much pressure right now with a new partnership—and the kids. My wife Mary and I have four kids, ages sixteen, seventeen, nineteen, and twenty-one. The youngest is driving her mother crazy with her constant back talk and "wild" ideas. And then the oldest just announced he's taking a year off from school to tour Europe. Mary, a nurse, works part-time—she says it's to help pay tuition and just because she wants to keep involved. I want her to quit. She wants me to spend more time with the family. I'm so torn. . . . Who comes first?*

Who's the "Sandwich Generation"?

As I use the term "sandwich generation," I mean explicitly those (like Alice and Don) who are under significant stress in midlife because of competing generational demands. The term is used to describe those persons who are pressed between the needs of their own children and the needs of their elderly parents. Women who delayed childbearing or couples who have had children later in life are often still raising their own children when elderly parents need support. Some are pressed from all sides with dependent younger children, dependent parents or in-laws, employment demands, older children who have returned home, and independent adult children who still appreciate some parental support.

Although the term "sandwich generation" does not exclusively describe baby boomers (those born during the birth explosion between 1946 and 1964), that category of 76 million Americans is demographically most represented in the term. It includes four out of every ten Americans and approximately nine million Canadians.

The Boomers Are Stressed!

The dominant lifestyle of the adult baby boomer revolves around the two-worker family. Most boomers have parents who are still alive, many of them sixty-five or older. They also have active, demanding children, often in their late teens and early twenties.

The combination of all these factors creates what some refer to as the sandwich generation. Visualize it by thinking of a submarine sandwich in which the meat and cheese in the middle (the boomer) is being squeezed by the pressure of dependent children, employment, parents, and the worry most will also have about their own retirement situation.

Gail Sheehy, in her book *New Passages: Mapping Your Life Across Time*, argues that people in the sandwich generation are truly entering new cultural territory. The longevity of their parents, the extended dependency of their own children, the high employment rate of midlife women—these competing stressors that their parents did not face come when the boomers are also facing midlife concerns related to their own aging process, retirement, and marital relationships.

Working Women

Increasingly, middle-aged women are employed in the labor force. In fact, trends indicate that with each successive age group, more and more women work outside the home. During the maturing of the baby boom generation, the size of the labor force skyrocketed as mothers went to work.

Women are also entering fields that used to be reserved almost exclusively for men. Women's participation in various trades such as building, forestry, telephone repair, and fire fighting has increased dramatically. Professional fields also employ growing numbers of women: at the present time, about 40 percent of medical school students, 40 percent of law school students, and 33 percent of MBA students are women.

Unfortunately, role models for today's middle-aged working women are hard to find in their mothers' generation. Who can teach them how to juggle the demands of work and family? Who can help them cope with the stress of providing for their children, assisting their parents, and keeping on top at work? Some women are pressed from all sides, overwhelmed with frustration, anger, stress, and unrelenting guilt. It's the "supermom" syndrome their mothers never experienced.

Midlife dual career couples also struggle with decisions of how much time to devote to the church and volunteer organizations. How much time is available to be a member of a school board, a church council, a denominational agency board? How does he or she weigh those decisions with the needs of the spouse, children, and parents? Related to this, of course, is the question, "How supportive is my spouse?" If one partner is very active in the church, the community, and career, how does he or she respond to the other's need for assistance in managing the home? For some men and women, given their family background and the era in which they were raised, these changes are difficult to make—even if they know they should occur.

"Boomerang" Kids

More and more sandwich generation parents can expect their adult children to return home. *"Grown children are like boomerangs—parents toss them away, but they just keep coming back." About 40 percent of young adults will eventually return to live with their parents; that's one in eight adults aged twenty-five to thirty-four. Among factors that contribute to this added stress for middle-aged parents are the high divorce rate, the decreasing number of young adults who finish their college education within four years after high school graduation, and*

9

the increasing number of high school dropouts who are less like-
ly to find permanent employment before their late twenties.

—"The Future of Households," *American*
Demographics, December 1993, p. 33

The divorce rate in the U.S. for first marriages is about fifty percent, for second marriages even higher. About one in eight divorced
adults live with a parent (*Youthworker Update*, January 1996, p. 5).
Therefore it is not unusual for a middle-aged couple to have a divorced
daughter who has returned home with two or three children, just at the
same time Grandmother has had a stroke. Neither should we overlook
the increasing possibility that a divorced son will receive custody of
his children and be faced with the role overload that often accompa-
nies single parenting.

Some middle-aged couples also have children returning home after college graduation to use home as a base while they search for a job.
Even after finding a job, or between jobs, some remain at home, considering it the cheapest board and room in town. They also frequently
expect Mom to take on earlier roles of cook, launderer, mender, and
nurse—even though Mom also has to be concerned about her employment status and Grandpa's deteriorating health. Dad may also assume previous roles, such as "on-call mechanic," while he's wondering
whatever happened to the more relaxed time he was enjoying with his
wife in the peace of their empty nest.

Aging Boomers

At the present time baby boomers are exploding into middle
age—the oldest of the boomers begin turning fifty in 1996. With that
demographic shift, baby boomers will begin to feel the effects of their
own aging process. "It's not just their sheer numbers that promise to re-
define what it means to grow old in America. As the best-educated,
most affluent, and healthiest generation in the nation's history, boomers are poised to rewrite the story of aging in America." Life expectancy for U.S. boomers is predicted to reach eighty-one for men and
eighty-five for women (*AARP Bulletin*, December 1995, pp. 1, 11). The
Canadian picture is similar, at least from the perspective of a war generation veteran who describes Canadian boomers as "better educated;
trim from rigorous exercise, surgical tucks, and low-cal high-fibre
diets; postponing marriage deep into their 30's or beyond; earning
more and casually spending more on things we considered luxuries . . . " ("The War Generation," Robert Collins, *Maclean's*, April 3,
1995, p. 47).

Listen to one boomer's story:

- *Hello, I'm Ralph. I'm forty-five and manage an engineering consulting firm. My wife is forty and is a full-time social worker. We both are very competitive and hope to advance in our careers. We have three children ages twelve, ten, and six. We're careful what we eat, and my wife and I both exercise two or three times a week. All of our parents are in their late sixties and in reasonably good health, although they aren't exercising on a regular basis. We're both convinced that by the time we reach retirement, neither Social Security nor Medicare will exist in their present forms. We believe that nursing home costs in the future will be a tremendous burden. We believe that aging is to a great extent the result of lifestyle, and we expect to age well.*

Ralph's right about the importance of lifestyle. People who are sedentary, smoke, and eat a lot of fatty food increase their probability of developing heart disease. The current sandwich generation is more aware than previous generations that a sedentary lifestyle can be devastating to one's cardiovascular system. The heart is a muscle, and like all muscles, it needs exercise. Consistent exercise also decreases the probability of obesity, which increases blood pressure and the probability of diabetes. The current sandwich generation may be the first generation that is sophisticated about LDLs (low-density lipoproteins which can cause plaque to form on the walls of arteries). Because diet is a major contributing factor to the development of high LDLs, boomers are more concerned than their parents about eating too much red meat, dairy products, egg yolks, and so on. Indeed, the Sunday dinner menu is changing—and Grandma isn't always happy about it.

Lifestyle decisions also produce changes in the musculoskeletal system. Members of the sandwich generation have been told again and again that to maximize their heart and lung capacity and maintain physical fitness they should walk, jog, bike, swim, or do any other type of aerobic exercise at least three times a week. Convincing Grandpa to join in might be a way to strengthen lungs and "hearts" (relationships) at the same time.

But while aging well is probably a goal of most boomers, aging will still bring its inevitable changes. Almost all will notice change in their sight, their hearing, and their skin. Many will notice a loss of hair, a loss of strength, dental problems, sexual dysfunctions, and neurological difficulties. Some will handle these changes with aplomb and confidently stride into middle age, while others will worry about their aging process and fear becoming old. Again, the sandwich generation is pressured by the simultaneous recognition of these changes in themselves while dealing with the effects of these changes in their parents' lives. (It isn't only the gray hair that's the same as Grandma's!)

Some women experience the added stress brought about by menopause. While most women go through this change without significant trouble, about 10 to 15 percent have a rather difficult time. They have trouble handling stress, just at a time when they are probably facing more stress than ever before.

Retirement Plans

- *Early retirement? You're kidding, Ralph—you're too young! But look at me. I'm fifteen years older than you, been around here a long time. Man, I'm counting the days—got the golf clubs all shined up and ready. And Norma's collected enough travel brochures to take us around the world. Take it from me, wise old Sam—those days come quicker than you think! Just keep dreaming, Ralph.*

Most middle-aged couples are thinking, planning, and fantasizing about their own retirement. Much of this fantasizing includes thoughts about travel, and more time for hobbies and other leisure-time activities. But often the burdens brought about by ethical, financial, and day-to-day decisions about the care of elderly parents can intrude and destroy the dreams and anticipation of these years.

Baby boomers will dominate the middle-age category for the next several decades. Public policy will encourage, even require, them to delay retirement. Canada and the United States can no longer afford to have their citizens spend one-third to one-fourth of their lives in retirement.

Some boomers will be the most affluent retirees in history, but many others in North America (about 25% in the U.S.) will face a retirement of financial risk. Some members of the sandwich generation worry about their own financial status in old age, wondering if government health-care programs will be available for them when they retire. Others worry about forced retirement, being cut loose early through corporate downsizing. Others are concerned about whether they are saving enough for their retirement years. Still others worry about persistent inflation, which over the course of thirty years could devastate their savings.

Often these concerns are compounded by what they see happening to their aged parents. The boomers look on as their parents begin to lose their estates to increasing medical costs that might include long-term nursing home care.

The boomers' economic future depends, in large measure, on whether public policies today—especially those involving Social Security, Medicare and pensions—will address boomers' diverse needs and enable them to look forward to a financially secure retirement and a lifetime of learning and productivity. It will also depend on whether the boomers take an active role in shaping and planning for their own future.

—"Boomers Will Find AARP a Resource in the Future,"
Horace B. Deets, *AARP Bulletin*, January 1996, p. 3

Sandwich generation members show a dualism about these issues. Public opinion polls indicate that they are pleased that their parents receive Social Security (Old Age Security in Canada) and Medicare, but they are deeply doubtful that they will receive comparable benefits. At the same time, many know that without these government programs their parents' financial situation would be extremely precarious. And they can't help wondering about their own future.

Midlife Crisis

After considering all these types of stress, we might conclude that midlife is in itself a crisis! The truth is that the overwhelming majority of Americans do not have a midlife crisis. Most persons who have a true psychological crisis in midlife have usually experienced psychiatric problems throughout their life. Despite the unfortunate reality of a few fifty-five-plus males running off with a younger woman, the occurrence is rare.

Still, tension between sandwich generation spouses may be a reality. Christian couples hope and strive for a oneness in marriage—a unity reflected in a deepening psychological, spiritual, and physical connectedness. Over the years, the partners have empathized with each other, worshiped God together, and fulfilled each other sexually. But the many kinds of stress the sandwich generation faces can have a negative impact on this desired oneness.

Just as the midlife crisis should not be overemphasized, the realities of added stress during midlife should not be minimized. Most people going through periods of stress can handle them adequately, but prolonged periods of stress can lead to significant anxiety, which can become debilitating both psychologically and physically.

Fortunately, in middle age many people are at the peak of their competence and ability to handle stress and responsibility. Many researchers believe that the hallmark of a healthy middle-ager is a feeling of being in control of a busy life and being involved in a broader world. Betty Friedan especially emphasizes that in the second half of

life people often realize that they are wiser, more affluent, funnier, and more mature than they were in the first half of life. (Boomers are probably hoping that others will realize this about them too!)
Welcome to the sandwich generation!

Suggestions for Group Session

Getting Started

Begin this session by introducing yourselves. Briefly explain your reason for attending these sessions on caring for elderly parents.

Perhaps you're feeling like the middle-aged Jewish father Tevye in *Fiddler on the Roof* when he said, "I don't remember growing older." David, the psalmist, expressed a similar sentiment in Psalm 103:15-16: "As for man, his days are like grass, he flourishes like a flower of the field; the wind blows over it and it is gone, and its place remembers it no more."

Begin → Facing the challenges of caring for our aging parents forces us to think about the brevity of life and about our own mortality. It seems like only yesterday that Dad was reminding us to "slow down" as Mom tucked a "care package" in the back seat, and we headed off to our new world of eagerly-awaited independence. Now we find ourselves *Trading Places* —we're the ones giving advice and providing care as our parents, much less eagerly, face a new world of decreasing independence. The following discussion questions and activities are designed to help you sort through the joy and pain this period in our lives can bring. In reality, we're all a part of the sandwich generation era— we're either one layer of the bread or the meat and cheese between the two layers. We can learn from each other and build stronger intergenerational ties.

Begin this discussion with a prayer to thank God for his faithfulness from the sunrise to the sunset of our lives and to ask for wisdom and strength to reflect his love to our aging parents and grandparents.

Group Discussion and Activity

1. Read 2 Timothy 1:5. If we can assume that three generations of Timothy's family were living at the time Paul wrote to the young man, Timothy's mother may have experienced some of the challenges of being "squeezed" in the middle. What benefit did Timothy receive from this intergenerational interaction? What blessings do we experience as we see our families span three, four, and even five generations?

2. Refer back to the stories of Alice, Don, and Ralph. Take a moment to share your own situations. What roles (spouse, parent, adult child, employee/employer, volunteer) are you juggling? How has the responsibility of caring for your aging parent(s) affected these roles? If you've not yet reached this stage, how might your roles change to accommodate the added role of caregiver?

3. Do you agree that the experiences of the sandwich generation are unique? Reflect on the family life experienced by your parents and grandparents. What particular challenges did previous generations, particularly your parents and grandparents, face in caring for their aging parents? How do they compare to today's challenges?

4. Which of the causes of stress discussed in this chapter put the most pressure on you and your family? (It's OK if you and your spouse choose differently—that makes a good topic for discussion later!) Break into smaller groups with those who share the same "primary" stressor. Share your frustrations and feelings and some coping strategies that you've found helpful. Bring your ideas for coping back to the larger group.

5. Think back to some of your favorite times with your extended family. You can probably still taste Grandma's fried chicken and corn-on-the-cob dripping with butter. And you wouldn't have thought of getting all choked up over Grandpa's cigars. Your dad probably stretched some unused muscles in a good game of softball with the kids, and Mom relieved her stress "gossiping" with your aunts over the dishpan. What's changed? Why all the emphasis on diet and exercise for the boomers—and their parents?

6. What influence do you expect the baby boomers to have on policies regarding their own retirement? What role can Christians play in assuring that the needs of every generation will be considered in the public arena? What can you do in your local community?

7. We do not know what the future holds, but we know who holds the future. How can this thought comfort us as we watch our parents age and experience the aging process in our own lives?

for oct. 7-

Closing

Read Psalm 90. Ponder these words from the notes for verse 17 found in *The NIV Study Bible*: "As you only have been our security in the world, so also make our labors to be effective and enduring—though we are so transient." Follow with a prayer that God will indeed bless the works of our hands as we care for our aging parents.

prayer

v. 17 May the favor of the Lord our god rest upon us — establish r work of our hands for us — yes — establish r work of our hands!

TWO

FAMILY DYNAMICS

- *Hello, I'm Mary. I'm a full-time homemaker and mother of three children, ages ten, sixteen, and seventeen. My husband Jack is a construction worker who moonlights as a security guard three nights a week to make ends meet. My father had a severe stroke last month—he's seventy-seven. Mom is trying to care for him at home, but she has high blood pressure and diabetes. She can be really demanding. My three siblings just assume I'll be available for Mom and Dad. They're all college graduates and work full-time, but it seems to me they aren't doing their fair share to help with Mom and Dad. Jack gets very angry about this—and about all the time I spend volunteering at church and at the kids' schools. I really want to be home, but I think Jack wishes I'd get a job. Everyone expects so much. . . .*

Who's Involved?

Intergenerational family dynamics become increasingly complex as the needs of aging parents multiply and intensify. The emotional strain affects the aged parents, the adult children, their siblings and spouses, and even the grandchildren and great-grandchildren. Ideally these extended family ties can be a built-in support system. In reality, they often become a tangled web of tension within and between the generations.

Although relationships are always changing, we can expect family relationships to exhibit some sense of continuity based on earlier family interaction. Families with a history of demonstrated love, respect for each other, and sensitivity to each other's needs will probably negotiate the tensions of change even during periods of intense stress. Families with a history of intergenerational conflict, substance abuse, indifference, and unresolved conflict will probably experience higher emotional tension and a resurgence of unresolved difficulties. Earlier scapegoats may again be the focus of familial rejection and anger. Old abuses may result in current verbal, physical, emotional, and/or financial abuse of aged parents.

Accepting Brokenness

Caring for our elderly parents can bring out intense feelings of anger, respect, love, frustration, guilt, or a combination of all of these. These feelings often intensify during times of crisis. Families may not have resolved all the problems they experienced during the child-rearing years; now when Mom or Dad are in a crisis, the old feelings can come galloping back. All families have experienced some brokenness in their intergenerational relationships. Understanding and accepting some of the reasons for our brokenness can lead to healthier relationships and strengthen family ties during crises.

Parental Abuse and Lifestyle

Some adult children have been the victims of emotional, physical, or sexual abuse. They are emotionally torn between past abuse and present obligations to an aging father or mother. From a human perspective, it is difficult, if not impossible, to give love when one has not experienced love.

In other instances, a parent may suffer from cirrhosis of the liver, the result of lifelong drinking binges. Adult children may be called upon to devote financial resources and much time, often at the expense of their spouse and children, to caring for such an alcoholic parent. The present psychological cost of caregiving is compounded by feelings of loss from the childhood years when the parent was often absent—at the bar or in a drunken stupor. Unresolved resentment can suddenly explode in decades-repressed torrents of angry words.

The biblical injunction to forgive is a basic goal for healthy relationships, but it is clearly very difficult for many adults to achieve. If we have been brought up by abusive or neglectful parents, a rhetorical assertion does not make the pain and hurt disappear. But God is certainly saying we must struggle against anger or grudges that will continue to disrupt relationships and corrode our own soul. Pastoral or professional counseling can be very helpful in the forgiving process.

Sibling Rivalry

No, we haven't switched topics. We're not talking about kids! Sibling rivalry for parental affection and attention often continues as long as the parents are alive. And it's not unusual for this rivalry to continue with the grandchildren.

These unresolved sibling rivalries may pop up again when families face decisions about caring for elderly parents. Old family hurts that everyone thought were "buried" suddenly make their reappearance. A "spoiled" brother you thought was always Mom's favorite is still excused by Mom when he fails to meet his obligations for care of the parents. Your "always-dependable" sister suddenly feels great resentment because she's the only one living in the hometown and now is expected to provide all of the care for Mom and Dad. Old feuds— about money loaned and never paid back, about college tuition paid or not paid, about gifts given or heirlooms promised—can add to the stress of deciding who contributes a "fair share" of resources for the care of the elderly parent.

Generational Differences

At times generational differences—either petty or significant— can also create tension in families. Each generation sees reality differently because their life experiences are influenced by the historical era in which they were raised. Generations disagree over church growth, liturgy, music, and structure; they argue about politics, the economy, and even family life. The Christian family struggles to understand and live out God's universals in a complex society.

Many intergenerational families argue over such things as dancing and alcohol at weddings, earrings in the ears of grandsons, the role of women in the church and in society, the way money is used, and dozens of other issues. Most Christian families resolve these issues with a sense of respect and often with a good dose of humor. But in other families the dynamics of parental authority intrude on what could otherwise be a civil discussion. Dad's voice rises in anger, or Mom sinks into dramatic silence because of different perspectives presented by the "younger generation, gone to the dogs." While in the best of worlds we may get wiser with age, some of us become old fools and ruin family relations with our angry, overly-controlling stance.

Our contemporary North American society also struggles with the broader generational conflict over the use of our collective resources. Unfortunately, the media attempts to create artificial conflicts between the old and the young. This attitude has not escaped the family circle.

- *I'm Harvey. I'm a thirty-five-year-old CPA and working on my MBA degree evenings at a local college. My wife is thirty-two and has a degree in accounting. She's studying to pass her CPA exam. We have two children, ages five and eight. We're very independent and career-oriented. We have a savings program in place for our retirement and for our children's college education. Our parents are in their early and mid-sixties, all healthy with a zest for life. Trudy and I resent older persons who are in need of government assistance because of failing health due to smoking, overeating and lack of exercise. We're afraid that we'll be overtaxed in the future to take care of self-centered, greedy geezers who are robbing the young of their economic future.*

What we need, both at home and in our larger society, is bridge-building between the generations. Instead of conflict between "canes" and kids, we need understanding of each generation's challenges and a willingness to share our resources for the good of all ages.

Role Reversal

- *When I was a little girl, my mother made me the prettiest clothes. Mom would fuss and say, "Janie, no grubbies today." I always loved the matching socks, and we'd giggle when my hair stood straight up with those fancy hair ribbons. Now I'm the one fussing. I cringe when Mom pulls on that old unmatched stuff from her closet. Seems like she just can't remember that I bought her some soft, pretty sweater and slack outfits. Feels like I'm the parent—it hurts!*

Some adult children struggle with a role-reversal process, in which a formerly revered and highly respected parent becomes dependent. They find themselves taking care of those who in the past were their caretakers. Suddenly, the one they always sought for help is the one that needs help.

Aging parents themselves may feel deep resentment and anger as they become more dependent. For most persons, a loss of dependence leads to a loss of self-esteem; and for many, to depression. Parents fear becoming a burden to their children.

There is no substitute for clear, honest communication between family members. Parents need to be able to discuss their anxiety, sadness, and frustration over the changes that are occurring. They must also be willing to listen to their adult children share their concerns about balancing time for caregiving with the responsibilities of rearing their own children, their marriage, their job, and their other responsibilities. Parents can quickly feel isolated when their adult children condescendingly make decisions for them and no longer include them in discussions about their own struggles in life. A fine line separates careful judgment about not "bothering" Mom with our own problems and simply concluding that Mom no longer has the mental or physical ability to be of assistance.

A family conference involving all of the adult children and the aging parents can be very helpful. Certainly past family dynamics will be part of the process, but a family conference can help prevent misunderstandings later. Decisions will be easier to accept if everyone has been included.

We probably all recognize ways that our present intergenerational family dynamics have been influenced by our past experiences. Most of us would agree that some interaction over the years has been good, some not so good. But relationships can change and grow. Families can reconcile, forgive each other, repent for past behaviors, apologize. Family members can ask God for a new beginning.

Strengthening Family Ties

The extended family in North America is a strong supportive resource for most members of the sandwich generation. Research shows that adults spend more time visiting blood relatives than they do visiting friends, neighbors, or coworkers combined. These are the "ties that bind." How can we strengthen these ties to hold us together as we face the challenges of caring for aging parents?

Touch

Physicians often tell us that touching helps the healing process. Most of us would agree that an embrace, a kiss, or a touch in a familial context denotes love and caring. We treasure being embraced by a spouse, a parent, a brother, or a child.

You may have heard the cliché, "What goes around comes around." Parents who were undemonstrative to their children will probably find in their old age that their children are undemonstrative to them. But we do have the power to change that pattern. If you come from a family that does not touch, begin by putting your hand on your parent's elbow—perhaps as you help Mom from a chair. It's amazing how "queenly" Grandma feels when a dashing young grandson repeats this kind gesture.

Be really outrageous—put your arm around Dad! Live danger-ously—kiss Mom on the cheek! Be a kid again—give Mom or Dad a great big bear hug just like your toddlers used to do. (If you need lessons, grandchildren give wonderful demonstrations!) Try these same expressions with your children and next thing you know, you've become a touching family.

A touch can frequently be more powerful than words. Words aren't going to make much of a connection with a parent in the later stages of Alzheimer's disease. Just watch, though, the reaction to an embrace or holding hands. Through touch the words of 1 Corinthians 13 come alive—we mean what we say, and our actions show it.

Reminiscence

Almost everyone enjoys reminiscing. We can learn about life dur-ing the depression, for example, and about our family history at the same time. Some families might want to consider videotaping or recording the conversation for future generations. Our roots lend sta-bility in a rapidly changing society.

Reminiscence can bring back happy memories of earlier times as we recall humorous events or the foibles of family members. Sometimes we can look back and share regrets over things we wish had not happened. Reminiscing can also help us deal with loss of loved ones as we go through the grieving process.

Since every generation has a different focus on life events, focus your reminiscence on things that meant the most to Dad and Mom. While country music or gospel music may not be your preference, it's doubtful that Mom and Dad have a nostalgic interest in tunes of the Beatles. Perhaps our grandchildren will be kind and insightful enough to ask us, "What did you really like about the Beatles, the Grateful Dead, or Peter, Paul, and Mary?"

Reminiscing says, "I care enough to spend this time with you. I'm glad we shared our lives together." Make it a regular part of your fam-ily times.

Gifts

Most of us have probably seen our Grandma's bureau drawer packed with boxes of lacy handkerchiefs and embroidered towels she was saving because they were too pretty to use. We can all recall the "sameness" of the neckties Grandpa got year after year. But in spite of that, most aging parents still enjoy receiving gifts from their family.

Gifts usually indicate a person was thoughtful enough to spend both the money and time to make or purchase something. A gift does not have to be expensive to make a point of love and consideration. A tape by a favorite musical group that Mom and Dad always enjoyed can show your thoughtfulness. A basket of flowers can speak volumes on your widowed parent's anniversary. The purchase of a magazine about gardening, or housing decor, or vacationing, or woodworking states rather well, "I thought of you when I saw this magazine." For parents who are financially struggling, sharing your newspapers and magazines is a thoughtful gesture. Grandma would be proud and pleased to receive a subscription to a particular magazine (maybe large print) for her birthday from a sensitive granddaughter. Or perhaps a season pass (complete with a grandson's escort service) to the local college basketball games would be just the way to show, "I love you."

Visits

Probably the best gift we can give is our time. For some of us, that means writing time into our busy calendars. We've all heard about the value of "dating" our spouses and setting aside time to spend with each child. Think of your parent's response if Dad or Mom could look forward to their own regular time with you—time to talk, to work together around the house or yard, to go out for dinner or for a ride to the old farm. Mark your calendar!

Visiting parents in their own home can be spontaneous too— dropping by for a cup of tea or to "smell the roses" together. Blessed are the grandchildren who can ride their bikes to Grandma's for homemade cookies and milk or walk to the old fishing hole with Grandpa. Many a rebellious moment has been eased during these times, and bridges built between the generations.

For many of us, those days of togetherness have stretched into miles and years between visits. Vacation time back home is often packed with catching up on what's happened to Dad and Mom. Letters and systematic phone calls, every Sunday or every other Saturday night for example, are time and money well spent. As the familiar slogan says, "Reach out and touch someone."

Family Gatherings

Older members of a family usually enjoy family reunions. Some families plan reunions at the same time and place every year so that every family member can put that date on his or her calendar. The elderly enjoy watching their descendants play and interact. It's an opportunity for younger members of the family to pay their respects to members of the older generation and for everyone to appreciate God's covenantal blessings.

Holidays can become a bit more problematic. Members of the sandwich generation are beginning to wonder which of their children will spend the holidays with them, with new in-laws, or even in a distant place alone. At the same time, they're concerned about if Mom and Dad can (should) still host the traditional Thanksgiving or Christmas gathering. The painting by Norman Rockwell of an aged, rather rotund, grandmother waiting in the doorway for family members to arrive for Thanksgiving dinner fills most of us with nostalgic feelings. Most likely there will be changes in the holiday celebrations as the family circle changes and ages, but certain family traditions can be preserved and treasured. Maybe Grandma won't cook the entire turkey dinner, but she might like to "supervise" the dressing and bring a batch of her homemade rolls or the favorite pecan pie. Grandpa might not remember "the little tyke's" name, but he can still don his "St. Nick" cap for a four-generation picture.

Is there a danger that we can become overly emotional about family relationships? Not really! It's probably better to err on the side of being overly sentimental than not being expressive enough. Strong family ties can be an emotional and spiritual legacy passed from one generation to another. That's why God places the lonely in families (Ps. 68:6).

Suggestions for Group Session

Getting Started

Open this session today by reading Eugene Peterson's contemporary version of 1 Corinthians 13:

Love never gives up.
Love cares more for others than for self.
Love doesn't strut,
Doesn't have a swelled head,
Doesn't force itself on others,
Isn't always "me first,"
Doesn't fly off the handle,
Doesn't keep score of the sins of others,
Doesn't revel when others grovel,
Takes pleasure in the flowering of truth,
Puts up with anything,
Trusts God always,
Always looks for the best,
Never looks back,
But keeps going to the end.

— *The Message*

24

As families face the realities of caring for aging parents, family dynamics can become complex and overwhelming. Just when we need each other most, we can be farthest apart. Peterson concludes his version of the well-known love passage with these words:

> *But for right now . . . we have three things to do. . . . : Trust steadily in God, hope unswervingly, love extravagantly. And the best of the three is love.*

Begin this discussion with circle prayers for faith, hope, and love to carry us through this period in our lives and to thank God for the best—his love to us and our aging parents.

Group Discussion and Activity

1. As your aging parents' needs increase, who is involved and affected by the decisions that must be made? Spend a few minutes sharing your family's answer to the question, "Who's involved?"

2. Look back at Mary's situation. What dynamics are evident in the interactions she describes? What suggestions would you make to change the situation into a more positive one for Mary and her family? (You'll probably find some interesting dynamics within your group as you struggle for solutions.)

3. If family relationships have been hurt by abuse, can these families forgive and forget at a time when they are experiencing a new challenge to their relationships? Why might this timing be so crucial?

4. Feeling a little embarrassed to admit that you and your siblings are still rivals? Share ways that you may have found to "kick this door open" for family discussion and get on with the business of helping your aging parents. "Spoiled little brother" may just have a different perspective of "big bossy sister" that will bring down the house and remind both of you that you were very loved.

5. What generational differences become "touchy" subjects at your family gatherings? How do members of the in-between generation handle conflicting ideas between the younger generation and aging parents about family values, religious views, and so on?

6. Look at Harvey's story. Do you share Harvey's and Trudy's concern about your economic future? What can be done to prevent this concern from becoming a social and political conflict between "canes" and kids? Does this conflict occur over use of church and denominational resources? Explain.

7. The reversal of roles with our parents comes on most of us unexpectedly. How can we communicate our feelings about this unexpected, and essentially unwelcomed, role? Try doing so from both the adult child's and aging parent's perspective.

8. Proverbs 17:6 paints a beautiful picture of family ties: "Children's children are a crown to the aged, and parents are the pride of their children." Think back to a time when you felt and saw this picture displayed in your extended family circle. Share briefly with the group or in small groups.

9. Several suggestions are given in this text for strengthening family ties. Which of those work well in your extended family? Which would you really like to expand? In what other ways does your family build on the bonds that have formed over the years?

Closing

Psalm 89:1 says, "I will sing of the LORD's great love forever; with my mouth I will make your faithfulness known through all generations." Use this verse to guide your closing prayer, or sing together "Great Is Thy Faithfulness."

THREE

SENIOR HOUSING

- *My name is Andrew. My father is eighty-six and very sharp mentally. But his heart condition and arthritis have really presented a problem in the last couple of years. He can't manage alone in his own home, but he refuses all offers of outside help. And he won't hear of any other living arrangement. My wife and I both work and can't keep ahead of the demands of two places. My sister tries to come about once a month, but it's a five-hour trip on weekends, and she's still got kids at home to worry about. What are we going to do?*

- *Hello, I'm Ginny. My mother's eighty and is determined to live alone in her own home, against her doctor's advice. She's used a cane, and sometimes a walker, since her hip replacement five years ago. I'm afraid she'll fall and no one will know. I know she doesn't cook much because she can't see well, and she hates to eat alone. I'm a single parent with two teenage sons, and we live twelve hundred miles away. I call Mom two or three times a week and just pray that my brother and his family will keep a close eye on her. They live just down the street, but. . . .*

"Aging-in-place" is a trend that's here to stay. According to a 1992 AARP survey of older Americans, 85 percent want to stay in their own homes. Only 13 percent of older people wish to move, usually to be closer to family. Also, an increasing number of elderly parents expect their adult children to take care of them as they age. So moving in with a family member is the second most popular housing option. The bottom line is that the majority of older Americans have done very little planning regarding their housing needs for later years. Their families are concerned about failing health and lack of enough money to meet the housing needs of their aging parents (AARP, *Understanding Senior Housing for the 1990's*, p. 3).

Housing Needs and Concerns

The AARP survey found that "older Americans face a number of issues regarding their housing as they enter their retirement years. These include the appropriateness (size, layout, etc.) of the housing unit; proximity to friends, family, and necessary services; home maintenance; housing costs that include utilities and property taxes in addition to rent or mortgage; and safety and security, to name just a few" (AARP, *Understanding Senior Housing for the 1990's*, p. 5). We'll take a closer look at some of these issues that especially concern the sandwich generation and their aging parents.

Accessibility, Safety, and Maintenance

Sooner or later, members of the sandwich generation will become aware that Mom and Dad are struggling to maintain their independence in their own home, probably designed for their younger years. When adult children analyze the future housing needs of their parents, they should think in terms of "what ifs." What will happen if Mom or Dad develop a severe heart condition, a broken hip, arthritis, or Alzheimer's disease?

Unfortunately, many families wait until a crisis happens with Mom or Dad before they deal with housing problems. The need for an accessible bathroom or bedroom on the main floor can become an instant crisis that needs an instant remedy. If Dad or Mom become less mobile or bedridden, what arrangements can be made to ease the care for the other spouse? Usually the answer to that question requires solutions that may take weeks or months to put into effect. Looking ahead, some families might want to consider building or remodeling to provide a bathroom or bedroom on the main floor.

Most accidents involving older adults occur in the house, and stairs are a major contributor to these accidents. Elderly adults frequently have trouble climbing stairs, and especially so while carrying baskets of laundry or other items. Saving trips to the basement can be as simple as moving a washer and dryer to a main floor closet or kitchen. Installing handrails on both sides of the stairs can provide added security for those "necessary" trips up or down stairs for Mom's "attic" search or to Dad's shop.

Some elderly parents find that their house and yard are simply too large for them to maintain. Rarely can an eighty-year-old woman (or man for that matter) put up a ladder extending to second-floor windows, wash those windows, and install storm windows. Related chores such as snow removal, lawn mowing, bush clipping, house painting, screen repair, and lawn fertilizing are persistent, but good intentions on the part of family members do not get them done.

Do busy sandwich generation members, with all their other responsibilities, have the time to do these chores? Frequently the responsibility for housing maintenance and yard work falls on the children living nearby, and they may resent the fact that other siblings are not doing their fair share of the work. Hiring these services out might be a solution. If parents are living on a very limited budget, the children can chip in to pay for these expenses. Or perhaps the children who live away might consider this their way to contribute their fair share.

Financial Concerns

Aging adults often find that as their housing ages with them, expenses for significant maintenance (roofing, a new furnace, new water heater, new siding, pest control, interior repairs, and so on) begin to take their financial toll. The problem is compounded by the fact that during this time of life, heavy medical expenses are also consuming a fair share of an often fixed income. Most elderly parents are unwilling to accept help from their children to pay for these expenses.

So, because it's easier to ignore the house than their health, some older Americans may see their own housing deteriorate along with an entire neighborhood. In some of these neighborhoods, as older persons die, their homes are purchased by speculators who then rent out the housing. Rental property is usually not maintained as well as owner-occupied housing. Deterioration begins. Not only do property values (a parent's assets) decline, but what once was a safe, viable community increasingly takes on characteristics of a slum. High poverty, high crime, and a lack of city services destroy any feeling of neighborliness or community. What once may have been a strong ethnic community—an Italian village, a Polish settlement, a Dutch enclave—with strong institutional identifications, becomes an area of angry,

29

alienated drug users and criminals. Mom and Dad then become frightened about going out at night, or even during the day.

In contrast, some older persons live in housing that has significantly appreciated. Again, the house may be too large or expensive to maintain; and parents may consider selling, to purchase a more affordable, smaller house. Older persons who are struggling financially can increase their financial security by investing the profit from the sale of their home, and decrease their housing expenses with a smaller home. Families may want to consult a lawyer or financial advisor regarding capital gains tax exemptions and other legal matters.

Whatever the situation, it's important for adult children and their parents to plan ahead. Will this house and this neighborhood be suitable for Mom and Dad ten or fifteen years from now? Often "now" might be the best economic and emotional time to make a move.

Support Systems

Researchers have shown that older persons rely on the informal network of family, friends, and neighbors first and most frequently. However, proximity to government services and help from other community organizations is another concern related to housing. Adult children need to ask, "Who can help if we aren't available?"

Many parents have accepted the reality of their children moving away for education and employment and never returning to the hometown. Some elderly parents are pulled to areas where most of their children relocated. Even though both aging parents and adult children may welcome the parent's relocation, both should expect a period of readjustment and even dependence of the older generation on the younger. Families will want to consider, "When is the best time to make this move?"

Other elderly people move for reasons of sociability. Research indicates that older adults who move into housing where most of the neighbors are of a similar age tend to increase their socializing. These neighborhoods of older people tend to have similar values and interests, similar life experiences, and therefore find it easier to relate to each other.

This type of community support can be a real comfort to adult children, whether it comes from Mom and Dad's old familiar neighborhood or from a new setting specifically designed for the elderly. The neighborhood coffee "klatch" crowd keeps a watchful and caring eye on each other.

Even though the overwhelming majority of older Americans stay in the area in which they lived out their working years, a few older Americans, a distinct minority, may move to a "better" climate. These older "snow birds" live in the South or Southwest in the winter and then return home to a northern state for the spring and summer. Many other older Americans travel in the South during parts of the winter months, but keep their only residence in the North. Adult children are frequently concerned about parents being able to locate emergency care when needed or maintaining consistent health care connections in their winter home. "Oh, I'll just wait until we get back" or "I don't like that new doctor" are excuses that can keep adult children awake at night. And a reminder to check the furnace and water the ferns will keep them running to the empty house.

Housing Alternatives

- *My name is Ray. My father and I have never been very close, and since Mother died, we really haven't gotten along too well. He's so moody and set in his ways, but I still feel responsible for him. His doctor has told him he shouldn't be living alone. After all, he's eighty-two and legally blind from diabetes. So he wants to move in with my family. My wife isn't saying a word one way or the other, but our two married children are against the whole idea. I'm not sure. . . .*

- *Hello, I'm Jessie. My mother really needs to move out of the old house where she and Dad have always lived. It's too big, and she just can't afford the upkeep. My two older brothers think she should come to live with me since I'm single and don't have a family. I've just made a career change and bought a condo about two hours from Mom. She won't know anyone here, and there's not much space. I just don't know. . . .*

Even though 85 percent of elderly people *want* to remain in their own homes, in reality only 35 percent of older Americans live alone. That means that almost two-thirds of parents of sandwich generation adults will face the decision of alternative housing. Even with the best accommodations for accessibility and safety, willing cooperation between family members for maintenance of the family home, adequate financial resources, and strong family and community support systems in place, adult children would be wise to discuss housing alternatives with their aging parents before the need arises.

Housing Choices: Independent Living
Condominium villages for the elderly are springing up all over the country and may present a good choice to those who can afford this option. The owners hold full title to their unit and joint ownership in

the common grounds. Snow removal and lawn care are provided by the management. In some cases services also include window washing, painting, screen repair, and so on. This frees elderly parents and adult children from major responsibility for upkeep. Often condominiums are located in newer, safer areas, and some provide additional security with restricted gate entrances and call boxes at the front door.

Many condominium communities also are good social environments for aging adults. Some have recreational areas and a common room for family reunions or resident gatherings. Others organize recreational events such as bus tours, lawn (cricket) tournaments, and shopping trips. Adult children are often amazed at the increased social life of their aging parents and find themselves having to "get on Mom and Dad's calendar."

Families considering the purchase of a condominium should read the "small print" of the purchase agreement carefully. Owners, through their representative board, will want the right to determine management fees, regulate recreational area use, and set policies for maintenance and upkeep of the common ground and housing units. Owners should have the right to determine quiet time, age segregation limits, resale agreements, and other policies. The right for resale should be clearly understood at the time of purchase. Giving attention to these legal matters can assure parents of an enjoyable retirement and relieve adult children of estate hassles later.

By the way, have you noticed that condo dwellers are getting younger? Who knows, the sandwich generation just might consider moving next door to Dad and Mom in their new setting!

Mobile or prefab housing may be a more affordable option for aging parents. This type of housing is usually exempt from real estate taxes, although it does demand a significant monthly service fee to the park owner.

Mobile home parks restricted for elderly families provide more opportunities for socializing with people of similar interests and increased safety and security. The one-floor design puts everything in a convenient and efficient location, but the limited space may mean less room to host large family gatherings and keep treasured things. Maybe Grandma's ready to give up the Sunday morning after-church coffee gatherings, but it's certain the younger generation will miss her cookie jar. And Grandpa may fuss about why that "handy old spade" was sold at the auction.

Before settling on the mobile home option, families need to investigate the long-term financial and social aspects of this choice:

- In some areas of the country, mobile homes may depreciate instead of appreciate in value.

- Sites can vary tremendously in regard to quality of services provided, charges for those services, and living conditions. More than once, a family has purchased housing for what they thought was an agreed-upon price, but a year or so later found that the service fee was raised significantly.

- In areas prone to tornadoes or hurricanes, it is wise to examine storm shelter accommodations.

- Parks that are open to families of all ages and income levels may be dominated by a particular culture or way of life. Before purchasing, it's wise to visit the park on different days and at different times. Is the park quiet? Are there loud parties on weekends?

Probably one of the best ways of getting a true picture of a mobile home park before buying into it is to visit with residents and get their opinions about services, fees, and environment. Talk to the local police department, too, about their perception of the crime rate and the frequency of police calls to the park. A prefab house in a well-run park with age segregation can provide many older parents an optimum housing alternative.

Lower income older persons might qualify for **government subsidized housing** in both the United States and Canada. Government subsidized housing is "means" tested. If a parent qualifies because of minimal income and assets, the government pays for the difference between a percentage of the elderly person's monthly income and the actual rent charge. Government subsidized housing for the elderly is built according to specifications that require minimal safety features like grab bars in the bathroom, emergency cords or buzzers in bedrooms and other areas, electric outlets higher in the wall rather than near the floor, and handrails in hallways.

Families will want to choose a location that is judged to be safe for the next several decades. The apartment should be located within walking distance of a shopping center or at least near a grocery store and pharmacy. Elderly people often check, too, for proximity to their church, the bank, and post office. Government subsidized housing is available in most parts of the U.S., but most units have a waiting list. Convincing parents to put their name on a list "just in case" might be a good idea and also gives the parents time to consider this option.

Another government subsidized housing program is referred to as Section 8 housing. In this type of housing, if older persons meet the guidelines in regard to income and assets, the government will subsidize their rental in privately owned rental units. The purpose of this type of subsidy is to enable impoverished older persons to have more freedom of choice in housing.

Government subsidized housing is at the center of intense debate in the U.S. in regard to its value, administration, and policies. The secret to successful government subsidized housing for the elderly is to have age-segregated housing located in a crime-free area. This type of housing has proven very successful for older citizens. It has enabled many impoverished older citizens living in crime-ridden neighborhoods to enjoy a safe haven in their later years.

Sandwich generation adult children can play a role in forming public policies that protect their own parents' choice and keep this option open for other needy elderly people.

European countries have introduced the concept of a **separate, self-contained, living unit placed adjacent to the existing home of a relative.** This type of housing gives the older person a greater opportunity to maintain independence, yet permits adult children to be readily available when the older person needs help. Some units are constructed so that they can be detached when the older person dies. Many variations on this theme could work in North America. A garage could be converted into an apartment, or a small efficiency apartment could be added to the home. This space could be rented out later or converted to an office or work area.

Maybe the idea of extended family under one roof will "come of age" with the boomers. It could give a new twist to the term "cottage industry."

Housing Choices: Semi-Independent Living

When we remind ourselves again that about two-thirds of elderly Americans do not live alone, we realize the importance of examining housing options as dependence increases. We'll explore a few of these choices based on a continuum of assistance needed.

One option that more and more families are considering is to keep Dad and Mom in their own home (perhaps the condo, mobile home, or apartment they chose at one point) and to obtain **in-home support services.** Homemaker and home health assistance is available through government agencies and private organizations. Meals on wheels, volunteer "taxi" service for doctor appointments, home delivery of groceries and prescriptions, visiting nurses—these and other community support networks can be lifesavers for aging parents.

Coordinating these services can still be a major responsibility for adult children, especially if they live some distance from their parents. Sometimes parents refuse to have strangers "meddling" in their day-to-day affairs. Other times, deep bonds of friendship form between the elderly and these "angels of mercy."

As Ray and Jessie shared with us, many adult children must consider the possibility of moving an aging parent into their own home. **Living with children** or other family members is the second most popular housing option considered by elderly people—second only to living in one's own home. "It appears that caregiving from family members is very much intertwined with older peoples' housing expectations" (AARP, *Understanding Senior Housing for the 1990's*, 1992, p. 54). About one-fourth of the persons surveyed by AARP indicated they would choose to live with family if they had to move from their present home.

The whole issue of accessibility becomes a consideration again, along with the often conflicting needs of two or three generations dealing with limited time, space, and energy. Who will give up a room for Grandpa? Do teenagers want to share the bathroom with Grandma? Who's going to look after Grandma while everyone works? Will siblings help pay for the expense of remodeling and routine living expenses? Can Grandma handle the hubbub of a coming and going household? Will Grandpa approve of the kids' friends? Will the sandwich generation couple give up their empty-nest time, maybe sacrificing any time together before or after their own retirement? The questionnaire *Under One Roof?* in Appendix A can help you consider some of the other questions and issues you might face.

Some older persons prefer to purchase into a **continuing-care community.** As the name implies, it means that aging parents may start out in an independent living unit. Then, if they become somewhat dependent, they may move into congregate living, where meals are provided. From there, if more debilitation occurs, they may move into supportive care and finally into nursing home care. The important point is that aging parents are guaranteed care the rest of their lives. Another advantage is that if one parent needs significantly more care than the other, it is usually provided on the "grounds," so the more independent spouse can visit easily.

Cost of buying into such a community can vary tremendously, depending on the quality and number of services provided. Families should investigate the institution's reputation for care and financial stability. It has not been unknown for such units to go into bankruptcy.

The continuing-care community can be a tremendous blessing for both aging parents and their children. No matter how far away adult children live, no matter how busy they may be, no matter what other obligations and responsibilities they may have, they can be assured that Mom and Dad will be taken care of by trained professionals. Older persons can have the security of knowing that they will not become a burden to their children.

Eventually, very few members of the sandwich generation are going to escape dealing with complex questions of what to do about suitable housing for Mom and Dad in their later years. Some of these adults will face questions about Mom and Dad at the same time their children are asking them for financial assistance—perhaps for a down payment on a home. They may also be struggling with questions about where to spend their own retirement.

The best way to avoid dealing with the stress such questions can create is to plan ahead. Although there are many alternatives for housing as one ages, making the choice during times of crisis can be traumatic. "Where would you like to live if. . ." might be a good topic for Sunday dinner discussion.

Suggestions for Group Session

Getting Started

Begin this session today by reading John 19:25-27 aloud. Ponder Jesus' concern for his mother during this time of great crisis. Think about Mary's feelings as she grieves and moves into John's home. Wonder about the changes this new responsibility brings in John's daily life.

Use a few minutes of opening prayer time to praise God for this example of caring for an aging parent. Seek God's wisdom and leading as we face decisions about our own aging parents and their changing housing needs.

Group Discussion and Activity

1. Split into small groups and share with each other the things you like best about your present home. Then imagine yourself at your parents' present ages. Could you still remain independent in the house you're living in now? What changes would you have to make?

2. Have your parents expressed the desire to "age in place"? Sometimes these desires may be expressed as offhand hints and other times as threats, daring you to think otherwise. How can you use these comments to open up conversation about the "what ifs" and help them think about possible alternatives?

3. Share some of the concerns you may already have experienced with your aging parents and their attempts to remain independent in

their own home. How can you be sensitive to their emotional ties to their home (and probably the home of your youth), and at the same time face the reality of their present needs?

4. The stories shared by Andrew and Ginny represent two ends of the proximity-to-aging-parents continuum. Living next door or far away both present challenges for the sandwich generation. Break into two groups to become advisors to either Andrew or Ginny. What would you do in either situation? Present your suggestions to the entire group for reactions.

5. Adequate and safe housing for the elderly is a national issue. How has your parents' community responded to the needs? If you are no longer a resident of that community, how can you mold decisions regarding elderly housing in your hometown?

6. What would you do if you were Ray or Jessie? How would your family answer some of the questions on the questionnaire *Under One Roof?* in Appendix A? Why do you think some cultures accept extended family shared housing as a way of life and others fear it?

7. If your parents needed to move from their present home in the next six months, what option would you choose for them? Share your "impromptu" decision with the group and offer suggestions to others to help them sort through their decision.

8. Maybe you know just the right realtor, mobile park owner, or home health service. Maybe you've already experienced wonderful support from a continuous-care facility. These networks can ease the burden during times of crisis. How can your group or others in your church share this information with other families who face similar decisions?

9. "Home is where the heart is." This motto may have hung on the wall in your parents' or grandparents' home. It's a reminder that houses are more than brick and mortar. How can this motto encourage you and your parents to "feel at home" wherever your parents live out their later years?

Closing

Home and hearth are important to all of us. Housing is considered a basic need for physical and emotional well-being. Jesus reminds us in his comforting words to his disciples in John 14:1-4 that home is important for our spiritual well-being too. Thank God today that Jesus went to prepare a place for our aging parents and that they have passed on this "estate" to us. Thank God that we "know the way."

FOUR

CAREGIVING AND CAREGIVERS

- *What a day! We spent the afternoon at the nursing home visiting Bill's dad, and it's the same old story. Dad complains constantly about the place—food, lights, noise, nurses—and Bill is such a softy. Bill thinks we should move Dad back home with us. I just don't think I can handle it. I'm afraid it will be just like it was when he was here before—no life of our own and all that tension. Besides, Dad's health isn't as good now either.*

- *Hello, I'm Sue. My mother still lives in her own apartment, and so far we're managing with home health care. But the doctor is advising my sister and me to think about nursing home care. Guess we should put Mom's name on the waiting list, but . . . I promised her I'd never put her in a nursing home. She's still mentally alert. Maybe I could take care of her in my own home.*

As we look at these scenarios and those in the previous chapter as well, we realize that our concerns about Dad and Mom's housing needs can very quickly become a much deeper concern about who is going to take care of them. For many families, the role of the family caregiver becomes a significant part of intergenerational family dynamics. Let's "walk in the shoes" of these families as we examine the expectations and challenges of caregiving.

Biblical and Cultural Mandates

The Bible clearly tells us that elderly parents are to be loved, honored, and aided. In 1 Timothy 5:4 we read, "But if a widow has children or grandchildren, these should learn first of all to put their religion into practice by caring for their own family and so repaying their parents and grandparents, for this is pleasing to God." And then verse 8 says, "If anyone does not provide for his relatives, and especially for his immediate family, he has denied the faith and is worse than an unbeliever."

These commands were given a long time ago, in a strikingly different culture, before Medicare, Social Security, Medigap insurance, government subsidized housing, nursing homes, and visiting nurses. What do these commands mean in the twentieth and twenty-first centuries? The Bible is not specific about how this honoring and caretaking is to be done. Certainly, though, God is telling us that we must be concerned about the well-being of our parents, grandparents, and other family members.

The Bible doesn't say that loving and honoring or caring requires that we take an aged parent into our home or pay for the cost of their nursing home care. Neither does the command state that children must allow themselves to be manipulated and controlled by overly authoritative parents. But the Bible clearly teaches that elderly parents are not to be ignored, shunned, or left to fend for themselves.

Our aging parents have devoted decades to raising their children. They've spent considerable amounts of money to provide necessities and often luxuries. They've listened to our problems and directed us in the Christian faith. They've struggled with the usual and unusual tensions and stresses, the inevitable universal aspects of parenting. God clearly expects reciprocal care from their children—including children whose parents were or are cantankerous, self-centered, or debilitated by Alzheimer's disease or depression.

Most North Americans, and surely the majority of Christians, believe that aged parents deserve the care and protection of their children. The biblical commands in Exodus 20:12, Leviticus 19:3, and Deuteronomy 5:16 are very clear. The moral absolute in these commands to honor and respect our parents is greater than any type of utilitarian emphasis or human selfish inclination. When our parents become old and frail, they still have the image of God, and they require our protection and love.

Even so, our obligations to our aged parents are not unlimited. We as adult children may want to be heroic in taking care of our aged parent, but we also must consider our own needs, strengths, and other obligations. While self-denial is clearly a part of the Christian life, we can practice a self-destructive martyrdom that only compounds a caregiving situation.

About 80 percent of older persons in America are cared for by family members. About 80 percent of those family members are women. Most older men are taken care of by their wives, and most older women are taken care of by their daughters or daughters-in-law. Overwhelmingly in our culture, women are expected to be the caregivers—ministering angels who willingly engage in radical self-denial for the good of other family members.

As we saw in the first chapter, the sandwich generation woman is caught between the conflicting needs of her spouse and children and the needs of her aging parents. And increasingly, sandwich generation women are taking leave from their jobs to care for aged parents. (Under federal law, any U.S. company with fifty or more employees must allow for at least twelve weeks of unpaid family leave. A *USA Today* report [7-19-95, p. B-2] estimated that the cost to companies of the lost productivity resulting from elder care responsibilities is about $17 billion a year.) Under these circumstances, it's understandable that the caregiving woman is often overwhelmed with feelings of inadequacy and guilt that she cannot meet all the demands and provide the level of care needed.

This is not to imply that all caregiving produces undue stress and inevitably results in anger, guilt, or depression. At times caregiving is satisfying and fulfilling. Meeting our filial obligations builds good feelings of self-worth. But what may be acceptable, even joyous, caregiving for one may be onerous and emotionally and physically overwhelming for another. We all have different strengths and weaknesses.

Most children genuinely want to be of assistance to their parents. Certainly, as we discussed in chapter two, our past intergenerational family dynamics can enhance or challenge our desire to help our aging parents. But even with the best of intentions, caregiving can be daunting, exhausting, and confusing. Parentcare, unlike childcare, usually does not have a happy ending. It's often a final chapter before death and can be accompanied by horrendous suffering and deterioration.

41

Stages of Caregiving

- *Hi, this is Jane. Have you talked to Mom lately? I called her last night, and she was so confused. All she talked about was Uncle Ned. 'Did you know he fell and broke his hip?' She asked me that three times. And she was all mixed up about when it happened and if he was still in the hospital. Last week when I talked to her, she had forgotten that you were coming home for the holidays. What's happening to her? Haven't you noticed?*

Caregiving usually goes through several stages. A realization that the older person is becoming either physically and/or psychologically debilitated usually signals the beginning. Children fear that something is "wrong" with Mom or Dad. This usually involves a discussion among family members about the extent of the changes that seem to be taking place. Sometimes the changes are obvious and dramatic because of a stroke, but at other times, as with Alzheimer's disease, the changes may be very subtle and elusive.

When it becomes obvious that changes are occurring, family discussions become more persistent. What is causing the changes? What is the extent of the changes? What can be done about them? Because these questions can often only be answered by physicians, adult children are faced with scheduling numerous clinic visits and making repeated decisions about who can accompany Mom or Dad. The various diagnostic processes usually produce a deluge of medical and insurance forms. At this point, if not earlier, questions arise about who will provide assistance to Mom or Dad. Who has the time? What needs to be done? Who has the know-how? This stage also often involves family discussions about whether or not everyone clearly understands the cause(s) of the changes. Grieving may occur as children experience the loss of a parent who was once independent and healthy.

Often before the questions are fully answered, the stage of continuing and constantly increasing caregiving begins. At first families may rely on support services delivered to the parent's home, or they may utilize these services in the adult child's home. Eventually, some aging parents will need assistance in bathing, toileting, feeding, and other activities of daily living. During this stage, balancing the needs of the dependent parent and the caregiver can present major challenges.

Finally, the stages of caregiving may end with the need to place Mom or Dad in a nursing home. Supportive family interaction is crucial during this stage. Probably no parent or adult child ever really wants this stage to come. But at what point can the caregiver(s) no longer cope? At what point do the responsibilities of the adult daughter become so manifestly burdensome that good intentions are no longer enough to resolve the problems of daily living for Mom or Dad? Intergenerational families must understand that all caregivers have a limit of energy, time, and psychological strength. Significant physical and/or psychological injury to the caregiver may occur if the situation continues unchanged. (We'll discuss long-term care further in the next chapter.)

Needs of Caregivers

- *It's been another thirty-six-hour day. Mom's getting weaker every day, and I've been up all night changing her sheets and doing laundry. Guess I fell asleep on the couch—didn't even hear Dan leave this morning. The house is a mess. I can't remember when I've cooked a decent meal. I'm so crabby, the kids don't even want to come for the weekend anymore. And I worry if I'll have a job when I get back—it's been two months now. God, where are you when I need you?*

Often caregivers are simply overwhelmed by the constant barrage of demands made on them. What are *their* needs? Where can they turn for help?

Help and Understanding from Family

Caregivers need tangible help from other family members. Often they must learn to ask for help and also learn to accept help when it is offered.

Family dynamics can become very murky at times. If an adult child is still trying to win the approval of an aged parent or attempting to provide most of the care as a means of shaming other siblings, accepting help can be difficult. If caregivers have been rebuffed when they've asked for help in the past, it's tempting to go it alone. But Christian families are encouraged to put aside these behaviors and develop a deepening awareness of the needs of the caregiver. Offer genuine and very specific help—a casserole for supper, money for a new perm, a day away with you in charge, a cleaning lady at your expense. Your keen and caring observations can add to the list.

Caregivers especially need understanding from family members when dealing with objectionable behavior on the part of the aging parent. Parents suffering from dementing illnesses are not responsible for what they say or do. Parts of their brain may be so destroyed by Alzheimer's disease or a stroke that they are no longer capable of normal adult behavior. They may say things that are hurtful, false, and even bizarre. Some parents may suffer from horrendously debilitating diseases such as Parkinson's Disease, and at the same time suffer severe depression. Other family members need to be sympathetic to the toll this takes on the caregiver who lives with this reality during repeated "thirty-six-hour" days. Just a simple "I'm sorry you have to hear this every day" from a sibling can lighten the load.

Family members also need to be aware of the potential for abuse of the caregiver by an aging parent. The abuse might be emotional: constant complaining, unreasonable demands, persistent fault-finding or berating. The abuse might be physical: scratching, hitting, kicking, even biting. Or the abuse might take on spiritual overtones as the parent issues a barrage of questions about her lot in life, his trust in God, or her fear of death. Accepting that these abusive behaviors can and do come from aging parents who were always gentle and loving and firm in their faith is difficult, but to deny their reality is to ignore and compound the caregiver's need for understanding and help. Again, a kind word, a hug, or a kiss on a bruised cheek from a spouse or child or sibling can comfort the caregiver.

✓   And sometimes that's not enough. Persistent abuse might be a warning sign that families need to consider long-term care.

Support Groups

Support groups can serve as an avenue for venting some of the frustrations caregivers experience. Caregivers often hate themselves or feel guilty when they have negative feelings or become impatient with their aged parent. Fatigue and stress tend to produce negative feelings. It is not unusual for caregivers to feel like screaming, "Enough, enough!" It's not unusual for them to want to run away from the situation or to wish for the death of the parent. It's not unusual for the adult children to become angry with an irrational parent—even when they know that the parent isn't capable of acting any other way.

✓   In the support group, the caregiver will discover that many other adult children have similar feelings and frustrations. It helps to know that other families struggle with the same problems. Support groups can also offer ideas, insights, and networks to agencies that are of considerable help in the caregiving process. Often they provide helpful literature and bring community resource people to the group meetings. Most community libraries, hospitals, clinics, or even the phone directory can connect caregivers with groups for caregivers, or with groups for families dealing with Alzheimer's, diabetes, cancer, strokes, and other debilitating diseases.

Stress Management

A major change in the health or behavior of a family member creates significant stress. Add this to the causes of stress we noted in chapter one, and it's no wonder that sandwich generation caregivers burn out.

Families of caregivers should be aware of the warning signs of excess stress. Changes in sleep patterns—insomnia, difficulty falling asleep—might indicate more than just a change in schedule due to the constant demands of caregiving. Chronic fatigue can be a sign of sheer physical exhaustion from the added physical care, but it can also indicate psychological exhaustion and a need for relief. Significant mood changes also signal too much stress. When a usually amiable person becomes irritable and angry, or a usually calm person becomes tense and hyperactive, it's time to relieve the pressure. Depression can hide behind apathetic or constantly morose attitudes or intense crying spells. An overly stressed caregiver may treat a parent in a rough, heartless, and demeaning manner. Some caregivers resort to alcohol or other drugs. When families recognize these signs of stress, it's time for intervention.

One excellent way to relieve stress is to exercise regularly. Family members can relieve the caregiver to allow specific time out for exercise. Knowing that a younger brother will drop by every day at a routine time can help the caregiver schedule a brisk walk or an aerobic workout at a health center. Perhaps an adult caregiver's married daughter can encourage Mom to walk with her every morning before Dad goes to work. Or giving a toddler a daily speedy stroller ride in the afternoon might be medicine for body and soul for the caregiver. Family involvement can overcome the excuse that the caregiver is too busy to exercise.

Rest and Respite

Members of the sandwich generation who attempt to juggle the needs of parents, children, and employment often sacrifice sleep to accomplish their long list of tasks.

Sometimes the aging parent is unaware of days and nights, or needs help during the night. A lack of rest eventually will lead to physical and mental exhaustion. Spouses and others who observe the day-to-day routine may need to insist that, "It's time to go to bed." "Power naps" in a quiet place, even at a neighbor's home, are no longer luxuries.

Caregivers must realize the limitations in their ability to give constant care. Taking time out each day to enjoy a television program or to read a favorite book or the newspaper is not a selfish indulgence.

Drinking iced tea with a neighbor in the backyard and sharing gardening secrets can provide relief from the constant pressure of thinking and talking about Dad's latest demand or the newest medication his doctor prescribed. Sharing a humorous comment Mom made about the lunch menu can ease the tension when supper isn't ready on time.

All caregivers need respite—a total break—from caregiving. They need periods of relief while someone else takes on the burden. Caregivers need time away to enjoy a night out with a spouse at a favorite restaurant, attend a concert or a church service, watch a grandchild's athletic event, plan a child's graduation party. They need time for laughter and joy, a relief from the grief and anger they are experiencing.

Intergenerational families will do well to recognize and respond to the needs of the caregiver. Often they can turn to the community for additional support.

Community Resources

Families overwhelmed with caring for their aging parents may be surprised to learn that for almost every problem, private or government agencies in their local or larger community offer a solution. However, awareness of and access to these services can prevent families, especially in more rural areas, from seeking this help. We'll highlight a few key resources available to most aging Americans. Canadian families will find a similar support system with slightly different names and programs. In both the United States and Canada, these community-based programs are proving to be vital for keeping the elderly in their own homes as long as possible.

Financial Assistance Programs

Most elderly North Americans receive some Social Security benefits. In the United States, elderly persons sixty-five and older may also qualify for **Supplemental Security Income.** This program, administered by the Social Security Administration, sets specific income guidelines and is designed to supplement the income of those elderly people (and children and adults with disabilities) who cannot manage on the limited income provided by their Social Security check. An estimated one-third of older Americans who do qualify have not applied for these benefits. Adult children who feel their parents might qualify should check with their local Social Security office.

Families might also wish to investigate programs such as the **food stamp program, energy assistance,** and **weatherization programs.**

These programs, administered by the Department of Social Services, are also based on income qualification guidelines.

Medical Assistance Programs

Social Security recipients qualify for **Medicare** insurance. Premiums are deducted from the recipients' monthly Social Security check and are adjusted annually to reflect inflation. Families can request a pamphlet from their local Social Security office, explaining what Medicare does and does not provide. Often adult children are surprised to find that Medicare does not pay for dental care, prescriptions, eye glasses, meals, or transportation (except for specific ambulance charges). Aging parents who can afford the premiums might wish to purchase Medigap insurance to pay for the charges not covered by Medicare. Families will want to shop carefully for these policies and compare costs and benefits.

Elderly recipients of Supplemental Security Income, and other impoverished Americans, also qualify for **Medicaid.** Income eligibility is determined by the Department of Social Services. Medicaid is a state/federal partnership. Each state, within broad federal guidelines, establishes eligibility and benefits, and funding is shared by the state and federal governments. This program, especially for those aging parents unable to afford Medigap insurance, can mean the difference between minimal and necessary health care.

Elderly veterans may qualify for health care programs administered through the **Veterans' Administration**. Area offices or veterans' hospitals can provide information about specific qualification requirements.

Information and Referral Services

The Department of Social Services, Adult Services can serve as a "first stop" when families are seeking support. As noted, the Department of Social Services administers several programs that can provide financial and medical assistance, and the agency frequently refers families to other needed services within their agency and the community. Every county in the United States provides these services through its Department of Social Services.

Strategically located geographical areas within the United States also have an **Area Agency on Aging** funded by the federal government. The Area Agency on Aging coordinates and contracts with other agencies to provide needed services to keep elderly people in their own homes. It is an excellent source of information about the numerous programs available in an area and can refer families to these services. When families call, they should describe the health condition of the parent and the type of assistance needed.

A national organization called **Elder Care Locator** can give information about community resources for older Americans anywhere in the country. The toll-free number is 1-800-677-1116. Adult children who live away from their elderly parents may find this service especially helpful for locating services in their parents' community.

Advocacy Services

A **community health nurse** from the Department of Health or a **visiting nurse** from the Visiting Nurses Association (or from a proprietary or nonprofit agency) can make an assessment of a parent's health and caregiving needs. Often they will review what services will be covered by Medicare and refer families to other services. Some will assist with the complex Medicare paperwork. Families may find the nurse's recommendations helpful if the time comes for long-term care placement.

Hospital **social workers** provide information and referral services to families who have hospitalized an aging parent. Because hospitals are under pressure to release patients as soon as possible, adult children must realize that the released parent may still need considerable care. The social worker, along with the medical staff, will also work with families when a parent's hospitalization leads to nursing home admission.

Private **geriatric care managers,** usually nurses and social workers, can be hired to act as advocates for elderly parents. They can provide a one-time assessment to determine the needs of the aging parent, recommend available services, and help families plan for future care. Some provide ongoing care or act as an emergency resource for respite care. These private geriatric care managers are usually very knowledgeable about community resources and also about the aging process and family dynamics. They are professional care providers, and their fees may range upward from $75/hour or more.

This brief review is not meant to provide an exhaustive list of available community resources. Families are encouraged to begin the process with one agency and to insist on referrals to other agencies that can provide the necessary assistance. The *Care Management Worksheet* in Appendix B at the end of this book may serve as a beginning assessment tool and a good focal point for family discussion.

Caregiving is more than an act of love. It's a decision-making process that requires ongoing communication and a delicate management of time, money, energy, and other resources as families seek to meet the needs of their aging parents. Caregiving is an intergenerational challenge. May we all be faithful servants.

Suggestions for Group Session

Getting Started

Begin the session today by reading two short passages: Mark 15:40-41 and Philippians 2:25-30. Note that "caregiving" is not a new concept. Picture the women lovingly taking care of Jesus' needs during his ministry and standing by, helplessly, as he died. Sense the sacrifice and physical struggle of Paul's "brother" as he helped Paul and stood in for others who could not be there. In both passages we see love in action, but not without stress and anxiety.

Spend a few minutes in silent prayer and thanksgiving that Jesus, the Son of God, came to earth to experience real human needs and the loving care of ordinary people like us.

Group Discussion and Activity

1. Read again the biblical mandate in 1 Timothy 5:4, 8. What do these ancient words mean to you and your family today?

2. How many decades have your parents devoted to raising children? What sacrifices did they make for you and your siblings? Is one's role as a parent ever finished? Explain.

3. Why are women, more than men, expected to be "ministering angels who willingly engage in radical self-denial for the good of other family members"? Can these cultural expectations be changed in your family situation as you care for aging parents? Share suggestions you have found helpful. (You might want to discuss these questions in separate male/female groups and then share perceptions and ideas as a whole group. Is this a gender issue in our society?)

4. Although the stages of caregiving presented in this chapter could seem overly simplified, they are meant to help you assess initial concerns. Using these stages and the *Care Management Worksheet* in Appendix B, do a quick evaluation of your aging parent's needs. (You may prefer to do this at home and use the worksheet to facilitate discussion with other members of your family.) If time permits, share your parent's major needs briefly with the group and describe the stage of caregiving you are facing right now.

5. Break into small groups and brainstorm ways to help the caregiver who described her "thirty-six-hour" day. What are her needs? Where can she turn for help?

6. Perhaps in the last session you thought of ways you could share information about resources you found helpful when dealing with the issue of housing for your aging parents. How could your church alert families to other helping agencies and programs in your community? What services could the church provide for caregivers and their families? (If your church is already involved in this type of ministry, how effective is the service offered, and how do families get involved in serving and being served?)

7. How can caregiving become an intergenerational act of love and service? Think of ways family ties can be strengthened as grandchildren and even great-grandchildren participate in the caregiving, even if from miles away. What models will the sandwich generation leave their children?

Closing

As you face the concerns of caregiving now or in the future, keep the words of 1 Peter 5:7 in mind: "Cast all your anxiety on him because he **cares** for you."

The words of the hymn below may be a favorite of your parents. This hymn was often sung by George Beverly Shea during the Billy Graham crusades. Use these words as your closing prayer today and perhaps read them or sing the song to your parents to comfort them.

His Eye Is on the Sparrow

Why should I feel discouraged? Why should the shadows come?
Why should my heart be lonely and long for Heav'n and home,
When Jesus is my portion? My constant Friend is He:
His eye is on the sparrow, and I know He watches me;
His eye is on the sparrow, and I know He watches me.

"Let not your heart be troubled," His tender word I hear,
And resting on His goodness, I lose my doubts and fears;
Tho' by the path He leadeth but one step I may see:
His eye is on the sparrow, and I know He watches me;
His eye is on the sparrow, and I know He watches me.

Whenever I am tempted, whenever clouds arise,
When songs give place to sighing, when hope within me dies,
I draw the closer to Him, from care He sets me free;
His eye is on the sparrow, and I know He cares for me;

His eye is on the sparrow, and I know He cares for me.

Chorus:
I sing because I'm happy, I sing because I'm free,
For His eye is on the sparrow, and I know He watches me.

—Text written by Civilla D. Martin (1868-1948)

FIVE

LONG-TERM CARE

Eventually many members of the sandwich generation will have to face the reality that Mom or Dad can no longer function independently and will need continuing nursing home care. Currently only about 5 percent of the elderly live in nursing homes. Of those admitted, about half stay less than six months. One in five will stay a year or more, and one in ten spend three or more years in a nursing home. It's estimated that almost half (45 percent) of people who turned 65 in 1993 will spend part of their lives in a nursing home (*Guide to Choosing a Nursing Home*, 1993, U.S. Department of Health and Human Services, Health Care Financing Administration, pp. 2-3).

The majority of adult children experience significant emotional stress when faced with placing a parent in a nursing home. If anything, families postpone this decision too long. Let's examine the emotional impact and quality of life and economics issues involved when considering nursing home care for our elderly parents. Then we'll discuss some challenges when placement does occur.

It's an Emotional Decision!

- *I knew when Mom broke her hip that the time had probably come. Still when the doctor said she couldn't go home. . . . The social worker was helpful, but I never realized there was so much involved with admitting someone to a nursing home.*

And to walk away and leave Mom there, crying, so alone. . . .
I suppose tomorrow her name will be on the directory at the
front entrance: Bertha Dykstra, Room 203. It all seems so
cold and impersonal. I'm sorry, Don, I know this isn't what
you wanted for Mom, but I just don't think we have a choice.

For an aging parent who is seriously debilitated, in need of skilled and continuing nursing, the nursing home may indeed be the best solution. Even so, the decision to place a parent in a nursing home usually arouses strong feelings in both the parent and the adult children.

Most older people do not readily admit that they believe it is time for them to go into a nursing home. They dread the thought of losing their freedom, of living an institutional life. They resent the idea of being bathed, fed, and put to bed at hours determined by nursing home staff and regulations. The thought of these changes often creates strong feelings of anger and anxiety in elderly people. They may lose their self-esteem and may become depressed. It is not unusual for parents to take their feelings out on their children or on the nursing home staff. Even in the most willing situations, everyone must expect a period of adjustment when an aging parent moves into a nursing home.

The most logically and medically sound reasons for nursing home placement may not erase the feelings of guilt on the part of the adult child. As we discussed in chapter four, the Bible instructs us to care for members of our own family. Adult children may ask, "Am I being selfish by placing Mom in a nursing home? Should I quit my job? Am I just unwilling to devote more time to a needy parent?" Some parents add to these feelings of guilt by reminding a child that they (the parents) took care of their own parents (the child's grandparents) until they died, and they never thought of nursing home placement.

The question of whether to place a parent in a nursing home also frequently involves sibling tensions and disagreements. Sometimes a sibling who lives farther away may not realize the intense demands for caregiving. Some families may fail to communicate along the way, so the decision may come as a surprise to some of the children. Other times, a crisis catches everyone unprepared for the sudden change, leaving the family confused and upset with any decision that is made regarding the aging parent.

Placing a parent in a nursing home is a very complex decision, one that involves tremendously powerful feelings. No one probably makes the choice purely on a logical basis. By planning ahead for the "what ifs," families can ease the stress involved and make a good choice of facility and location.

It's a Quality-of-Life Issue

- *Susie, did you know they were bringing me here? Why didn't somebody ask me what I thought about it? You just tell your mother she better think about getting me out of here. I want to go home—no reason why I'm just sittin' around here with all these sick people. Next thing you know, you won't even want to come to see Grandma anymore. This old folks' home's no place for a young woman like you with the babies.*

The U.S. Department of Health and Human Services publication, cited previously, describes the quality-of-life issue so well: "When people enter nursing homes, they don't leave their personalities at the door. Nor do they lose their basic human rights and needs for respect, encouragement, and friendliness. All individuals need to retain as much control over the events in their daily lives as possible" (*Guide to Choosing a Nursing Home*, p. 3).

Knowing some of the key provisions of federal nursing home reforms that went into effect in October 1990 can help families evaluate care. The law provides that nursing homes must

- train nurse's aides.
- conduct a comprehensive assessment of resident's needs within two weeks of admission.
- allow residents the right to choose activities, schedules, and health care consistent with their interests and needs.
- provide a safe, clean, comfortable, homelike environment.
- provide the necessary care and services that enable residents to maintain their highest practicable level of physical, mental, and social well-being.
- prevent arbitrary transfer or discharge and provide reasonable advance notice if a resident must be moved.

In addition, the legislation provides specific rules that nursing homes certified by Medicaid and Medicare must follow. These rules relate to residents' rights regarding referrals, admissions, accommodations, room assignments and transfers, policies regarding financial matters, care services, physical facilities, residents' privileges, and the assignments of medical staff and volunteers. For example, residents have a right to obtain their mail unopened, a right to private conversation, a right to discharge themselves, and a right to confidential treatment. The right to confidential treatment is virtually an absolute right. No one working with nursing home patients may discuss their care or behavior with persons outside the nursing home. Residents and their families must be allowed and encouraged to talk to nursing home administrators and staff about their concerns.

Federal law requires each State Agency on Aging to have an Office of the Long-Term Care Ombudsman. Although the ombudsman cannot recommend one particular nursing home, he or she visits nursing homes on a regular basis and can provide information from the latest survey report on a specific facility. He or she can report the number and nature of complaints against the facility in the past year and the results of investigations into these complaints.

State health departments also publish an annual report on the performance of nursing homes certified for Medicare or Medicaid. The report must be posted at the nursing home. Ask the administrator or the local ombudsman about any identified problem and what has been done to correct the situation.

If your family is not forced to make an emergency decision, you may want to visit several nursing homes to determine which one best meets the needs of your elderly parent when and if dependence increases. Levels of care can vary all the way from independent living with on-call nursing staff available, to assisted living with varying degrees of care provided, to skilled nursing care twenty-four hours a day. The *Nursing Home Checklist* in Appendix C is a helpful tool to assess the quality-of-life and care a particular nursing home offers. It can also be used to evaluate the care your parent is already receiving and serve as a focal point for discussion with the nursing home administration and staff.

Of course, it is your responsibility to see that your parents maintain an acceptable quality of life and receive quality care. However, adult children can become overly demanding. Obviously, your parent is the focus of your concern. To nursing home staff, your parent is one of a large number of residents needing continuing care. Staff often care for patients who are demented and who strike out, curse, and refuse to cooperate. They too feel the stress of caregiving. Still, if you believe that your parent is not receiving adequate care or is in any way being abused, you must not hesitate to complain to the administration or to the local ombudsman program.

It's an Economic Issue

- *Yes, Don, I've investigated every possible alternative. We'll have to sell Mom's house. Her nursing home care is costing $2500 a month. I've already used up her savings and the small life insurance policy Dad left her. No, Mom doesn't really know what's happening. I'm thankful we did the power*

of attorney, but it's just so overwhelming . . . and so sad
. . . their life savings . . . gone.

For most families, financing nursing home care is a major concern. Families fear that with the passing of time, nursing home payments will slowly but surely eliminate the bulk of the parent's estate. Some parents go into a nursing home with great sadness, knowing that none of their lifetime earnings will be left for their children.

Families may consider various options to protect some of their parents' assets. The process of determining how much parents can give to children and how they can best save their estate in the case of nursing home placement becomes very complex. Adult children may want to consult an attorney who specializes in this area. There also are moral considerations of distributive justice. How much is one morally obligated to pay for one's own care? To what extent may one morally attempt to preserve a lifetime estate for children and grandchildren?

Nursing home placement is also a major expense for the government, and increasingly the government is becoming less and less willing to pay. The U.S. government now has a thirty-six-month look-back period. This means that if parents attempt to give away their estate (or portions of the estate) within thirty-six months of nursing home placement, this act will be considered an attempt to purposely eliminate one's own responsibility to pay for nursing home costs. The government then has a right to confiscate funds or assets that were given away within the thirty-six-month look-back period prior to nursing home placement. In addition, the federal government is requiring that every state develop a plan to obtain payment from the estate of any nursing home patient for whom the government made Medicaid payments. Clearly in the future, with the growing number of older persons, the government will attempt to have families make, to whatever extent possible, full payment for nursing home placement.

Adult children and their aging parents currently finance nursing home costs in four basic ways. (Information about these four means is abstracted from *Guide to Choosing a Nursing Home*, pp. 11-15.)

- Personal Resources
    About half of all nursing home residents pay for costs from their personal resources. Depending on the length of stay and the level of care required, families may see their parents' assets disappear. At that point, adult children will want to check on financial eligibility requirements for Medicaid.

- Medicaid
    Medicaid pays for skilled and assisted nursing home care (care

57

that is above the level of room and board but less than skilled care). Individuals must meet income and asset eligibility requirements which vary from state to state. Regulations also govern transfer of resources by either spouse thirty months prior to nursing home admission. The "spousal impoverishment" provisions allow a spouse still living at home to protect a certain amount of income and assets. Families will want to contact the local Medicaid office early in the placement process and also verify that the nursing home selected is Medicaid-certified.

- Medicare

    Under very specified circumstances, Medicare hospital insurance (Part A) will pay for skilled nursing home care. Medicare only pays for skilled care following a hospital stay of at least three days. Released patients must require daily skilled nursing or rehabilitation services that must be performed or supervised by professionals. Medicare will pay for at least some of the costs for up to one hundred days per benefit period. For the first twenty days, the resident pays no deductible or coinsurance; beginning with the twenty-first day, residents pay a coinsurance. Coinsurance rates are calculated each year. Medicare residents must be placed in the section of the nursing home that is Medicare-certified. Nursing homes are required to give residents notice of noncoverage at the time of admission or when skilled services are no longer needed.

- Private Long-Term Care Insurance

    Some private "Medigap" insurance policies supplement Medicare coverage for care in a skilled nursing facility. However, these policies generally cover very little long-term care at home or in a nursing home, usually covering only deductibles, coinsurance, and long hospital stays.

    Families might want to consider purchasing long-term care insurance. This type of insurance covers nursing home care and may also cover home care. Because costs and benefits vary widely, careful shopping for "Medigap" and long-term care insurance is essential.

    The financial implications of nursing home placement for our aging parents can be overwhelming. Meeting the tremendous costs and dealing with the complexity of the various programs add to the stress adult children face. As caregiving transfers from the home and family to the nursing home and professional staff, seeking help from community agencies continues to be important. No one needs to struggle through this process alone.

Mom's in Room 203

- *It's so good to have you home, Don. Mom seems to be adjusting to the nursing home. Some days I don't think she realizes where she is. Most of the time she just sits in the chair and looks out the window. She does enjoy the music—lots of church groups come to sing and visit. Mom's in Room 203. I hope she'll recognize you . . . she's really changed since you saw her last.*

Once Dad or Mom have been placed in a nursing home, adult children and their families are faced with a new challenge. Visiting a more dependent elderly parent and maintaining a meaningful relationship in a new setting can be difficult. Much of the interaction will depend on the mental and physical condition of the parent and on past family dynamics.

As we noted in chapter two, demonstrated affection is very important to aging parents.

A touch, kiss, or embrace can speak volumes. Family members can give and receive love by embracing an elderly demented mother who still has the capacity to feel the warmth of that embrace. Less privacy and previous family dynamics may make these expressions seem awkward at first, but it's worth the effort. We'd do well to rewrite the bumper sticker: "Have you hugged your mom (dad) today?"

Conversation should be consistent with the parent's level of cognitive ability. If Mom or Dad has lost short-term memory, it's easier to reminisce about the past. Long-term memory is the last to be lost. Some parents who cannot remember who visited them ten minutes ago can recall vividly what happened in their eighth-grade class. They seem to relive life's simple pleasures—the smell of the summer pasture, the cool breeze under the huge oak trees in their backyard, the cry of the first newborn lamb. It's good to pull out these topics to encourage a parent to communicate and to stimulate the mind and senses. "Remember that baby colt we had, Dad?" or "Mom, remember how I dragged that old quilt around—the one Grandma made?" Questions like these can make an afternoon visit enjoyable for the entire family.

Bringing family photographs to the nursing home often results in a happy nostalgic look at the past. It also can give children a chance to label photographs and identify unrecognized relatives. Sometimes old magazines can elicit a smile and a memory from an aged father or mother as they share personal stories of World War II, the depression, or a local event. Most elderly parents enjoy talking about their family history. Children and grandchildren can gain some valuable and interesting insights into their own past. Families might want to record these oral stories as Dad or Mom share who immigrated, who served in military service, who died of what condition and under what circumstances, and other strong memories from the past.

Most older persons go through a period of evaluating their spiritual heritage. Some elderly parents question their own faith, doubt God's promises, or become indifferent. They will need our encouragement and assurance that God is still present in their lives. God tells us in Psalm 71 that older persons have a responsibility to talk about his truths to future generations, and God tells us to honor and to listen to our parents as they share what they believe about his grace and faithfulness—and their own struggles. It's so easy sometimes to feel that Grandpa's "preaching." Maybe he doesn't have the best delivery, but he's sure got a great message!

Reading aloud to an elderly parent or grandparent is a thoughtful gesture. Favorite books, poems, devotionals, and cards received from relatives and friends can open up new topics for conversation and bring cheer and comfort to a parent with failing vision and concentration. Think of the pleasure a young reader could share with Grandma as they enjoy a first grade read-aloud book together. And it might surprise you how well Grandma remembers her phonics!

You might volunteer to do correspondence for your aged father or mother. Perhaps Mom or Dad still enjoys sending cards to friends and relatives. Bring a special date calendar, a box of cards, and a book of stamps to help them keep in touch. Sending out cards or written expressions of concern is one way your parent can continue to be a contributing member of the Christian community.

Some nursing home residents can play table games such as *Monopoly*, checkers, cards, or *Scrabble*. Unless there is significant intellectual decline, our elderly parents are often bored and ready and willing to participate in a "rousing" game of *Monopoly* with the grandchildren. These fun times can develop or renew strong bonds between grandchildren and grandparent. For young children a game of *Old Maid* may rejuvenate Grandma and bring volumes of laughter from the grandchildren.

Many parents in a nursing home enjoy being taken out for special events: a holiday dinner, a Memorial Day parade, a Christmas party, and so on. They also enjoy a ride in the country, dinner at a favorite restaurant, or a walk in a nearby park. Children can take turns doing this and schedule outings as regular events on Mom or Dad's calendar. The anticipation of these good times is almost as exciting as the times themselves.

"That's my favorite!" Watch Mom's eyes light up when you bring a dozen of her favorite chocolate or butterscotch cookies, or hold your nose as Dad opens a jar of pickled herring. These thoughtful gifts remind Mom or Dad that you've paid attention over the years; you know them well and you love them more. The smell of roses, the sounds from an old band, the warmth of a flannel shirt, the violet color of a new sweater—these little reminders can turn a sad disposition into the jovial personality that kept things rolling at your home.

Adult children and grandchildren who live some distance from the nursing home can devote more time when they come for visits. They can also telephone periodically, send cards and amusing clippings from their newspapers, and occasionally send a special gift (food, flowers, games, books, clothes, or a subscription to a favorite magazine). In addition, they can show due gratitude to siblings who are close and who visit on a more regular basis.

The success of these ideas and numerous others that could be tried will depend on the mental and physical condition of your elderly parent and on the history of your family's dynamics. Nursing home placement often exacerbates feelings that we have developed over the course of decades. If we can forgive injuries from the past and build on the goodness we shared, we can develop a new depth of relationships within our family that will serve as a source of comfort and strength now and for the future.

Suggestions for Group Session

Getting Started

Read Psalm 71 together. Experts on the psalms think it very possible that David wrote this psalm in his old age as a prayer for God's help to face the afflictions of aging and to praise God for his faithfulness. Note especially the psalmist's request in verses 9 and 18, and his reflection on God's care throughout his life in verses 5-6 and 17.

Use the opening prayer time to thank God for his faithfulness to your aging parents and to share prayer requests that God will meet your parent's specific needs.

Group Discussion and Activity

1. Think back to your earliest experience at a nursing home. Perhaps you visited an elderly grandparent or other relative, or maybe your youth group or club did a community service project. Share your

impressions, your anxiety, your sense of duty or joy. Do these early experiences influence how we view nursing homes today?

2. If you have not already faced the decision of nursing home placement, have you been able to discuss this topic with your parent(s)? If you have already completed this step, what suggestions can you share to help others face the "what if"? Why is "nursing home" such a dreaded topic for most of us?

3. Can you identify with Bertha Dykstra's children? Share some of your own personal emotions and experiences as you look ahead (or reflect back) to the day Mom or Dad is assigned a room number.

4. As you think of the quality-of-life issue for nursing home residents, what one or two things would you consider most important for your parent's well-being in a nursing home? Can legislation or even your own investigation of a particular nursing home assure that these aspects will be a part of the quality-of-life offered your parent? (You might wish to refer to the *Nursing Home Checklist* in Appendix C.)

5. What role can you play as your parent's advocate? How will you balance your loving concern for your parent with the realities of staff demands, your parent's disposition, your own availability and ability to discern quality care?

6. Should the government expect families, aging parents and their children, to make full payment for nursing home placement? How aware are you of the actual costs for nursing home care and of the resources your parents may have available?

7. Break into groups of two or three and visit Room 203 with Don. Proverbs 17:22 sets a good tone: "A cheerful heart is good medicine, but a crushed spirit dries up the bones." What suggestions for visiting given in this chapter might work in Don's situation? Which ones have you tried successfully with your aging parent(s) or would you be comfortable trying? Share other experiences that have made visiting your parent or others in a nursing home especially rewarding for you and brought comfort and cheer to them. Share a few of these ideas with the larger group.

Closing

Watching our parents age and thinking about our own aging can weigh on our hearts and minds. Sometimes a different perspective can lighten our load. Let these words from a children's book do just that.

When I am old with you, Grandaddy, I will sit in a big rocking chair beside you and talk about everything An old dog will sit by my feet, and I will swat flies all afternoon. . . . When I am old with you, Grandaddy, we will play cards all day underneath that old tree by the road . . . and we won't mind that we forgot to keep score, Grandaddy. When I am old with you, Grandaddy, we will open up that old cedar chest and try on all the old clothes that your grandaddy left you. We can look at the old pictures and try to imagine the people in them. It might make us cry . . . but that's OK. . . . Grandaddy, when I am old with you we will take long walks and speak to all the people who walk by us. We'll know them all, Grandaddy, and they'll know us. At the end of our walk, when we're tired, Grandaddy, I will sit in a big rocking chair . . . beside you.

—Excerpted from *When I Am Old with You*
by Angela Johnson, illustrated by David Soman.
Text © 1990 by Angelo Johnson.
Reprinted by permission of the publisher,
Orchard Books, New York.

Psalm 37:25 says, "I was young and now I am old, yet I have never seen the righteous forsaken. . . their children will be blessed." Close with silent prayers asking God for a renewed sense of his presence and peace for yourself and your aging parent.

SIX

DEATH AND DYING

- *Remember the stories Grandma used to tell? She often told about her own grandmother's death. I think she was just a little girl then, and it must have been quite an experience for her. She said they put the casket right in the living room (the parlor, they called it then). Her grandpa helped move the pump organ to make room. Her mother hung a black wreath on the outside door to "announce" the death. And the family and neighbors all came. Everybody wore black and talked in hushed voices. Seems strange now, doesn't it? But sometimes I wonder. . . .*

Increasingly the sandwich generation will have to deal with the death of their parents and grandparents and with the reality of their own mortality. Perhaps we all wonder if we are better prepared to face death than our grandparents were a generation ago.

At the beginning of the twentieth century, life expectancy was less than fifty years. Death was usually swift from accidents; infections such as diphtheria, typhoid, pneumonia; or from other illnesses that today can either be cured by surgery or by medications. In those days death was "seen." Family members often died at home. It is not unusual for older relatives to have vivid memories of their aged parent dying. They may recall the smile they saw on their parent's face at the moment of death. Some witnessed a seeming heroic struggle between life and death before a parent died. Dr. Sherwin B. Nuland in his book *How We Die: Reflections on Life's Final Chapter* points out that death was a member of the family. Death was accepted as part of the cycle of life: birth, growth, maturity, aging, and then death.

Today the probability is much higher that death will involve a prolonged process of dying, often in an institutional setting. Members of the sandwich generation struggle with difficult questions involving quality-of-life versus sanctity-of-life in a society trying to determine who should receive, even who's "worth" receiving, medical care.

Death and Dying Issues

- *I've been reading a lot about power of attorney and living wills lately. Seems like there's some disagreement about what people should do. Guess I thought our wills were good enough. Maybe Mom and I should talk to you about all this once. Wish we knew more about it.*

It is becoming increasingly more important for aging parents to discuss their final wishes with their adult children. It's no longer enough to think of just the legal matters surrounding the estate. Intergenerational families will want to investigate options such as power of attorney, living wills, organ donation, and prearranged funerals. Incidentally, these issues present important questions for sandwich generation adults to share with their own children too.

Durable Power of Attorney and Living Will

We've heard much in recent years about withdrawal of life-support systems, doctor-assisted suicide, and the right to choose. These are difficult moral issues often requiring decisions during significant periods of crisis. These concerns can be addressed by signing an *advanced directive*, a document that sets out guidelines for our future care. The two most common types of advanced directives are the durable power of attorney for health care and the living will. Since state laws and legal documents will vary from state to state, families will want to seek legal counsel.

Adults, especially aging parents, should appoint a person to be their health care "agent" or "attorney-in-fact." This person will make health care decisions for the parents when they are no longer capable of making the decisions themselves. The agent must make the choices the parent would have made. In some states, the power of attorney document has two parts, one assigning the agent to make financial decisions while the parent is still living but unable to make these decisions, and the other giving the agent power to make health care decisions.

A living will is a document that gives precise instructions to your physician as to the circumstances under which you want life-sustaining treatment to be withheld or withdrawn. Adults can request that no heroic methods will be used to keep them alive and may specify their wishes regarding extensive chemotherapy, artificial feeding and hydration, and resuscitation. They may direct medical staff to administer whatever painkillers are necessary to control their pain so that they can die with dignity. In most states, directions in the living will apply only to terminally ill patients, and some states restrict the withdrawal of artificial feeding and hydration.

Since much has been written about the pros and cons of each directive, families will want to examine both of these options carefully. It's very important that families clearly understand what they have chosen and how these documents will influence their decisions during the dying process. It's also important to share these documents with the family physician.

Families will benefit from discussing the spiritual aspects of these directives as well. Dr. Nuland, in his book cited earlier, points out that dying is often a messy, agonizing process devoid of dignity. He warns that physicians have been trained to save life and that some will pursue expensive and exhaustive medical treatments to prolong life. Often older persons die in intensive care units, tangled in a "spider web" of wires and tubes. Christians can indicate that an expedited end to life is acceptable. Advanced directives can serve as another expression of a parent's faith, as they demonstrate that they are not afraid to die. The dying process is just the last chapter in the Christian's life journey to eternity.

Organ Donation

One of the last great acts a Christian can do is to have his or her own organs donated to benefit a living person. Most people in need of organs are placed on a waiting list, due to the shortage of matching donors.

There are many misconceptions about organ donation:

- Organ donation will hasten the death of the patient.
- The body will be so disfigured by organ removal that it cannot be shown in an open casket.
- Hospital staff will no longer give desired care if they know organ removal is planned.
- Hospitals will sell organs to make a profit.
- The family will be charged a large sum of money for organ removal.
- Organ donation will interfere with funeral plans.
- Most major religions strongly oppose organ donations.

All of these statements are false.

It is true that timing is important in organ donation. It is also true that after age seventy organs may be less acceptable for donation than are the organs of younger donors. Certain infectious diseases may also prevent organ donations. Medical histories will enable families to make this decision with the advice of their physician.

Donors should make their wishes explicitly clear to their families. Some states allow donors to indicate their wishes on their driver's license. Families may be asked to consider organ donation at the time of death even if parents or spouses have not indicated they wish to be a donor.

Prearranged Funerals

Funerals provide a cultural ritual, enabling relatives, friends, church members, and others to come together to give condolences and expressions of support to surviving relatives. It is an opportunity for organizations and individuals to send flowers or donate to a designated charity. The funeral offers an opportunity for the church, represented by the pastor, to give a presentation on the meaning of life and death. For some it is an opportunity to give a eulogy for the deceased.

A prearranged funeral can assure elderly parents that their funeral plans and expenses will not be a burden to their children. Increasingly, older adults are prearranging payment for their funeral, purchasing a burial plot and marker, and planning the details of the funeral service. If there is no preplanning of the funeral, surviving spouses and adult children are faced with making these difficult decisions at a time when they are dealing with a deep feeling of loss and often when they are already exhausted from the dying process. Although there is no evidence that the majority of funeral directors are unscrupulous, preplanning can help families avoid having to make decisions under undue emotional stress. The American Association of Retired Persons has an excellent pamphlet titled *Prepaying Your Funeral*, which can help you and your parents work through this process.

Support Systems

As we've discussed the challenges of caring for our elderly parents, the need for support continues to surface. Even the most strongly bonded families need a network of support during the final stages of a parent's life. We'll look at a few key support systems that can make a real difference for families who are coping with death and dying. (*The Care Management Worksheet* in Appendix B lists many other resources that offer support.)

Hospice Care

In 1967 Dr. Cicely Saunders started a hospice movement in England to help people in the dying process. Since then, the hospice movement has spread throughout the world. Most metropolitan areas in the U.S. and Canada now have hospice programs, and many smaller communities also provide significant hospice support.

Hospice programs attempt to give people supportive care so that they can continue relationships with their close relatives and friends until they die. The dying person, the family, and the medical profession openly and honestly accept the fact that death is near.

The hospice philosophy is carried out in several different ways. Some hospitals designate certain rooms as hospice rooms for the terminally ill and provide beds and other services so family members can share in the care and dying process. Other programs are closely affiliated with a hospital, but provide a separate residence setting near the medical center for the patient and family members. Some hospice programs also provide at-home care. Hospice organizations can assist family members with some of the routine physical care and provide specialized support for both the patient and the family from social workers, nurses, physicians, pastors, and trained volunteers.

Medicare covers many services under hospice care if the patient's physician certifies that a patient is terminally ill (a life expectancy of six months or less). *Hospice Under Medicare*, an excellent pamphlet explaining the hospice program and Medicare coverage, is available from the National Hospice Organization, 1901 North Moore Street, Suite 901, Arlington, Virginia 22209 (phone 703-243-5900). Your local chapter may have this publication and other information about licensure, standards, and so on.

Private long-term-care insurance may also cover hospice care. According to the National Hospice organization, HMOs are not required to provide hospice care, but those receiving monthly Medicare payments must inform Medicare recipients about Medicare-certified hospice programs in the area. The hospice patient may continue to receive other HMO benefits not covered by Medicare.

Hospice provides a loving environment where family members can say goodbye. Families facing the death of an aging parent or other terminally-ill loved one may want to consider this option. Dying at home or in a homelike setting can help all of us to accept death as a part of life and to treasure the faith and trust shared by an aging parent and grandparent.

Grief Support

- *My dad died very suddenly and unexpectedly. Mom grieved that she never got to say goodbye. We all missed his stubborn, independent spirit and realized how much Mom depended on him. I think the hardest part was seeing Mom so alone and lonely.*

Sandwich generation members often find themselves dealing with their own grief while attempting to assist a parent through the grieving process. Helena Lapato in her book *Widowhood in an American City* reports that research shows children can best support grieving parents by helping them regain their independence. In reality, many adult children tend to give Mother too much continuing assistance at the time of Dad's death.

Lapato also warns against making major decisions too quickly after the death of a spouse. Mom may argue that the house reminds her too much of Dad, and through her tears, beg to sell it. Adult children can encourage Mom to work through the grieving process first and then make decisions about keeping or selling the house. Frequently, after more reflection, Mom realizes that she likes the neighborhood, has friends nearby, and is comfortable in a house in which she has lived most of her life. Some widows are amazed at the abilities they uncover and become proud of their independence. Some widowers are equally amazed that they can learn to keep house and even enjoy cooking.

Lapato found that for many widowed persons, the best person to help them in the grieving process is someone who has gone through the same process. Many local communities and churches have support groups for those who have lost loved ones. The American Association of Retired Persons has founded the Widowed Persons Service to meet the practical and emotional needs of widowers and widows. There are over two hundred Widowed Persons Service organizations throughout the U.S., and they serve some seventy thousand newly widowed persons each year. Sandwich generation children may need to alert a grieving parent to these groups and possibly even make a connection with someone who attends. Taking the first step is always the hardest.

The Church's Role

- *What are we going to do with all this food? And look at all the cards and memorials! Mom, I'd forgotten how caring your church has always been and how much these people meant to Dad. What would we have done without them this week and all the time Dad was sick? What a blessing they've been to you.*

In the face of death and dying, the Christian community is tied together by shared faith and shared fellowship. Christians can meet the social needs of those who are dying. Too frequently, dying persons are isolated; they feel abandoned and forgotten by the church community. The caring church can develop an organized program of pastoral and elder visiting and counseling. The church family can also bring meals, provide friendship, run errands, and offer other assistance such as child care for grandchildren, help with cleaning and laundry, and transportation to the hospital. Families coping with terminal illness can often benefit from a more organized program of assistance that provides specific and scheduled assistance.

The church can take an active role in preparing its members to confront the health care and death and dying issues facing society today. The sandwich generation, simply because of numbers, will be the dominant influence on important decisions in both the political and medical arenas about the rationing of medical care, the permissibility of physician-assisted death, the indiscriminate use of medical technology, and the North American cultural orientation toward death and dying. The current sandwich generation may be the generation that insists that we do away with the dying charade and begin to talk openly about death and dying. They may also be the generation that insists no one should die in pain. Christians—baby boomers and others—need an opportunity to sort through these issues with other Christians and seek a biblical basis for their decisions.

The Christian community can provide, through preaching, teaching and sharing, affirmation of death and dying as part of God's plan to bring us to eternity. John Suk's *Dad's Dying* (CRC Publications) provides a sensitive "glimpse into the dark valley of death and the glorious resurrection beyond." It would provide excellent follow-up discussion material for your group.

As we conclude this six-session discussion on caring for our elderly parents, it's likely that many of you are already *Trading Places.* Some of you anticipate that role in the future. Whether we are elderly parents, adult children, or the younger generation, we can rejoice and testify: "I am not my own, but belong—body and soul, in life and in death—to my faithful Savior Jesus Christ" (*The Heidelberg Catechism A1*).

Suggestions for Group Session

Getting Started

Read Genesis 27:1-4, Joshua 13:1, and Joshua 23:1-2, 14. These brief passages remind us of two well-known Bible characters who, realizing they had come to the end of their years, took time to set their affairs in order. *The NIV Study Bible* notes for the passages in Joshua give us a special perspective on this stage of our lives: "The heavenly King . . . begins the administration of his realm (13:1). Joshua . . . delivers a farewell address recalling the victories the Lord has given, but also reminding the people . . . their mission remains—to be the people of God's kingdom in the world (23:1-16)." Life and death are both part of the journey to eternity.

Begin the session today sharing with prayer partners. Thank God for his plan for our lives and for our parents' lives from birth to death. Ask for his guidance as we carry out our mission to be his people.

Group Discussion and Activity

1. Are members of the sandwich generation less prepared to face death and dying than their grandparents, or even their parents? What experiences in your own life may influence your personal response to this question?

2. Are intergenerational families becoming more open to discussing death and dying issues? How can the sandwich generation take the lead in bringing topics like living wills and prearranged funerals to the attention of both the older and younger generations?

3. What *advanced directives* do you want to leave for your family? (Break into groups of two or three, or discuss this question with your spouse or family member attending.) Why do you feel the way you do about these last wishes? How could you communicate these feelings to your aging parents for their benefit and to your own children?

4. Do you know anyone who has donated or received an organ? Would you consider it? How can this be "one of the last great acts a Christian can do"? (Eleanor Grotenhuis gives a moving personal testimony of the blessings of this act of giving in her book, *Song of Triumph*, 1991, Baker Book House.)

72

5. Some people feel it's morbid to prearrange one's funeral. How do you feel about this practice? What benefits could it have in your family situation?

6. What hospice services are available in your parent's community? Have you considered serving as a hospice volunteer? How can the hospice program help intergenerational families to better accept death as a part of life? What caregiving challenges might be presented?

7. The sandwich generation continues to feel the "squeeze" during the grieving process. How can members of this middle generation cope with their own grief, help the younger generation face death (probably for the first time), and at the same time support an aging parent during this difficult new experience? Break into small groups and share some ideas for coping and resources to tap.

8. What is your church doing to prepare its members for the reality of death and dying and the hope of the resurrection? What would help you the most? Share these ideas with your pastor and church leaders.

9. Romans 12:13 and 15 remind us: "Share with God's people who are in need . . . mourn with those who mourn." What would families in your church do without the support offered during times of illness and death? If you have never received this support, you will undoubtedly find your family overwhelmed with the outpouring of love. If you have been a recipient, what did your family appreciate most? What suggestions can you give to make this ministry even more supportive?

Closing

✓ *There is a time for everything,*
and a season for every activity under heaven:
a time to be born and a time to die. . .
a time to weep and a time to laugh,
a time to mourn and a time to dance. . .
a time to love. . .
a time for every deed.

Ecclesiastes 3:1-2, 4, 8, 17

✓ *There is a time for* Trading Places,
a time of caring for our elderly parents.

Close this final session by praying together this paraphrased passage from Philippians 4:4-7:

Help us to rejoice in you, Lord, always; to say again: Rejoice! Let our gentleness be evident to our aging parents. Lord, you are near to them and to us. Help us not to be anxious, but in everything, by prayer and petition, with thanksgiving, present our requests to you. And may the peace of God, which transcends all understanding, guard our hearts and our minds in you, Christ Jesus.

SUGGESTED READING LIST

Aikery, L. *Dying, Death, and Bereavement*. Boston, MA: Allyn and Bacon, 1991.

Apter, Terri. *Secret Paths: Women in the New Mid-life*. New York: W.W. Norton Co., 1995.

Bartlett, D. and J. B. Steele. *America: Who Really Pays the Taxes?* New York: Touchstone Books, 1994.

Belsky, Janet K. *The Psychology of Aging*. Pacific Grove, CA: Brooks/Cole Publishing Co., 1990.

Bouma, Hessel III, and others. *Christian Faith, Health and Medical Practice*. Grand Rapids, MI: Eerdmans, 1989.

Buckinham, R.W. *The Complete Hospice Guide*. New York: Harper and Row, 1993.

Burnell, G. M. *Final Choices: To Live or To Die in an Age of Medical Technology*. New York: Insight Books, 1993.

Butler, R. N., Myrna I. Lewis and Trey Sunderland. *Aging and Mental Health: Positive Psychosocial and Biomedical Approaches*. New York: Macmillan, 1991.

Callahan, D. *Setting Limits: Medical Goals in an Aging Society*. New York: Simon and Schuster, 1987.

Climo, Jacob. *Distant Parents*. New Brunswich, NJ: Rutgers University Press, 1992.

Dychtwald, K. and J. Fowler. *Age Wave*. New York: Bantam Books, 1990.

Enck, R. E. *The Medical Care of Terminally Ill Patients*. Baltimore, MD: Johns Hopkins Press, 1994.

Forword, Susan. *Toxic Parents: Overcoming Their Hurtful Legacy and Reclaiming Your Life*. New York: Bantam Books, 1989.

Friedan, Betty. *The Fountain of Age*. New York: Simon and Schuster, 1993.

Grotenhuis, Eleanor. *Song of Triumph*. Grand Rapids, MI: Baker Book House, 1991.

Hampton, John K. *The Biology of Human Aging*. Dubuque, IA: W.C. Brown, 1991.

Hayes, Christopher L. *Women in Mid-life*. New York: Hayworth Press, 1993.

Hooyman, N. R. and H. A. Kiyak. *Social Gerontology: A Multidisciplinary Perspective* (second edition). Boston: Allyn and Bacon, 1991.

Hospice Under Medicare. Arlington, VA: National Hospice Organization, 1992.

Kart, C. S. *The Realities of Aging: An Introduction to Gerontology*. Boston: Allyn and Bacon, 1990.

Kermis, M. *Mental Health in Late Life: The Adaptive Process*. Boston: Jones and Bartlett, 1986.

Lapato, Helena. *Widowhood in an American City*. Cambridge, MA: Schenkman, 1979.

Lustbader, W. and N. R. Hooyman. *Taking Care of Aging Family Members*. New York: The Free Press, 1994.

McGurn, Sheelah. *Under One Roof: Caring for an Aging Parent*. Parkridge, IL: Parkside Publishers, 1992.

Moody, H. R. *Aging: Concepts and Controversies*. Thousand Lakes, CA: Pine Forge Press, 1994.

Nuland, Sherwin B. *How We Die: Reflections on Life's Final Chapter*. New York: Random House, 1994.

Prepaying Your Funeral. Washington, D.C.: American Association of Retired Persons, 1989.

Rabins, P.V. and Nancy L. Mace. *The 36-Hour Day*. Baltimore, MD: Johns Hopkins Press, 1991.

Riekse, Robert and Henry Holstege. *The Christian Guide to Parent Care*. Wheaton, IL: Tyndale, 1992.

Russell, Cheryl. *The MasterTrend: How the Baby Boom Generation Is Remaking America*. New York: Plenum Press, 1993.

Sheehy, Gail. *New Passages: Mapping Your Life Across Time*. New York: Random House, 1995.

Smedes, Lewis. *Forgive and Forget: Healing the Hurts We Don't Deserve*. San Francisco: Harper, 1984.

Smith, H. I. *You and Your Parents: Strategies for Building an Adult Relationship*. Minneapolis, MN: Augsburg Press, 1987.

Smoke, Jim. *Facing 50: A View from a Mountain*. Nashville, TN: Thomas Nelson, 1994.

Suk, John D. *Dad's Dying: A Family's Journey Through Death*. Grand Rapids, MI: CRC Publications, 1991.

Understanding Senior Housing for the 1990's. Washington, D.C.: American Association of Retired Persons, 1993.

Zal, H.M. *The Sandwich Generation: Caught Between Growing Children and Aging Parents*. New York: Insight Books, 1992.

APPENDIX A

QUESTIONNAIRE: UNDER ONE ROOF?

You and your family can use this questionnaire to think through some of the concerns you might have as you consider moving an elderly parent into your own home. If possible, involve all those family members who will be affected by this decision in the discussion. You might want to add other questions to fit your situation.

YES	NO	
☐	☐	1. Is a separate bedroom available for your parent?
☐	☐	2. Will someone in the family need to give up a room for your parent?
☐	☐	3. Does the room provide space for daytime activities (reading, watching television, visiting, crafts)?
☐	☐	4. Is a bathroom available near the bedroom?
☐	☐	5. Will the bathroom be shared with others in the family?
☐	☐	6. Is the bathroom equipped with grab bars?
☐	☐	7. Is the bedroom accessible to other areas of the house (no stairs or long hallways)?

☐   ☐   8. Will your family and your elderly parent both maintain some privacy?

☐   ☐   9. Will your parent require a quiet environment most of the time?

☐   ☐   10. Will other members of the family be able to continue their regular activities in the home?

☐   ☐   11. Will your parent require assistance with tasks of daily living (dressing, bathing, eating, walking, and so on)?

☐   ☐   12. Will you be able to leave your parent home alone?

☐   ☐   13. Will your parent require extensive caregiving?

☐   ☐   14. Will your parent's usual routine (mealtime, bedtime, activities) interfere with your family's routine (or lack of a strict schedule)?

☐   ☐   15. Will your parent require a special diet?

☐   ☐   16. Does your parent relate well to your children and grand-children?

☐   ☐   17. Will your parent interfere in your child-rearing responsibilities?

☐   ☐   18. Will your parent attempt to develop a controlling relationship with you?

☐   ☐   19. Will your parent enjoy your friends and people you normally have in your home?

☐   ☐   20. Will you welcome your parent's relatives and friends into your home?

☐   ☐   21. Will your parent contribute to the expenses?

☐   ☐   22. Do your siblings agree to the financial arrangements?

☐   ☐   23. Do you and your spouse agree that your parent should come to live with you?

YES   NO

☐   ☐   24. Are your children supportive of the idea of your parent
                            moving in with you (and with them if they are still at
                            home)?

☐   ☐   25. Will your parent be happy in your home?

Space, accessibility, privacy, caregiving, finances, and intergenerational relationships are all important considerations. Creative problem solving and loving respect for each other can probably relieve many of the areas of concern, but everyone should expect a period of adjustment. Only you and your family can decide if moving your parent into your own home is the right decision.

CARE MANAGEMENT WORKSHEET

Directions: Check the items in the column on the left which describe your parent(s) now. Use this assessment to determine what services Dad or Mom need and to identify community resources available to assist you and your family.

This tool can serve as a helpful focal point for a family conference and for meetings with medical personnel and other service providers.

	My Parent	Services Needed	Resources
☐	really needs to get out and do something.	**Socialization/ Volunteering**— Programs designed to provide an opportunity to socialize with peers or to offer service without compensation	Nutrition sites, senior centers, daycare, friendly visitors, senior companions, YMCA/YWCA, city recreation department, Retired Senior Volunteer Program, AARP Talent Bank
☐	can do light housecleaning but needs assistance with heavy tasks.	**Chore Services**— Window washing, mowing lawn, roof repair, minor housing repair	Local social services, area churches, youth groups, neighborhood clubs

My Parent	Services Needed	Resources
☐ has some legal matters that need attention.	**Legal**—Assistance with matters pertaining to law	Legal counsels for the elderly, local bar association, Legal Aid, adult protective services, banks
☐ is grieving over the death of a loved one.	**Bereavement Support**—Dealing with the normal grieving process	AARP Widowed Persons Service, THEOS, National Association for Military Widows, local support groups through churches and funeral homes
☐ cannot drive or use public transportation. Taxicabs are too expensive.	**Transportation**—Special transportation for older persons	Private transportation, transportation for people with disabilities, Red Cross, city elderly transportation services. (Some offer service to outlying rural areas.)
☐ is unable to remain in his/her present housing.	**Housing**—Special housing options are available to the elderly	Retirement community, public housing, foster home, intermediate care facility, nursing home, skilled nursing facility, house sharing, group homes, American Association of Homes for the Aged
☐ needs help with food preparation and/or housekeeping and/or laundry.	**Homemaker Services**—Non-medical service to help an older person remain in the home	Social service agencies, private homemakers, Red Cross, Visiting Nurses Association
☐ needs assistance with personal care (bathing, dressing, grooming, toileting).	**Home Health or Personal Care Aide**—Personal and basic health care provided by a specialist	Private home health companies, Visiting Nurses Association, Red Cross, private nurses, community health nurses, social services agencies
☐ doesn't eat right.	**Nutrition**—Nutritious meals provided at home or group setting	Home-delivered meals, Meals on Wheels, weekend meals programs, senior nutrition sites

My Parent	Services Needed	Resources
☐ cannot be left alone during the day.	**Friendly Visitors or Intermediate Care Facility**—Volunteers who visit with the elderly or a facility which provides constant supervision	Adult daycare, live-in attendant, social service agencies, foster homes
☐ needs special services for physical limitations and impairments.	**Services for People with Disabilities**	Disease-specific organizations, veteran's organizations, civic organizations, local agencies for disabilities
☐ has health care costs which are unbelievable.	**Healthcare Cost Containment**— Reducing cost of quality health care	Medicare—Social Security Office, Medicaid— Department of Social Services, local insurance companies
☐ is depressed, suspicious, and/or angry all the time; just sits.	**Mental Health**— Evaluation of psychological stability (also see Complete Geriatric Evaluation below)	City Mental Health Department, geriatric social workers, crisis intervention unit, psychiatric hospitals, Alzheimer's Disease and Related Disorders Association
☐ is acting strange. Could he/she be senile?	**Complete Geriatric Evaluation**— Medical, psychological and social testing of older person	Doctor's evaluation of nutritional habits, health, medications to rule out possible physical illness; mental health testing to rule out depression; neurologist's diagnostic tests; Dementia Resource Center, Alzheimer's Disease and Related Disorders Association
☐ really needs 24-hour supervision even though he/she fights it.	**Private Nurse or Nursing Home**— Homes for the elderly offering 24-hour medical supervision	Private nursing organizations, local ombudsman, homes for the aged, local office on aging, hospital social services, American Association of Homes for the Aging

85

My Parent	Services Needed	Resources
has a terminal illness and wants to return home instead of dying in the hospital.	**Hospice**—Medical and social services designed for terminally ill patients	Visiting Nurses Association, American Cancer Society, Hospice Association, local hospital social services department, local churches

Directions: Check the items in the column on the left that describe the feelings of any family member involved in caregiving. Use this assessment to evaluate the needs of the caregiver and resources available to help. Sharing this evaluation with other family members can begin a discussion of how the family will cope as an aging parent's care needs increase.

I Sometimes Feel	Services Needed	Resources
overwhelmed. I have so many unanswered questions about aging and services for the elderly.	**Information and Referral**— Provides knowledge of particular services and recommendations of places providing those services	Local office on aging— Department of Social Services, Area Agency on Aging, case manager for elderly, city information and referral, Elder Care Locator (1-800-677-1116)
I honestly need to share my feelings with someone who would understand.	**Counseling/Support** —One-on-one consultation or meetings with other caregivers who share problems and coping skills	Support groups for caregivers of the elderly, pastoral counseling, city family services, social service agencies
other family members are not helping enough.	**Family Meeting**— Meeting of relatives to discuss responsibilities for elder care	Family service agencies, private therapist, case managers, social workers, family therapist
my caregiving responsibilities are negatively affecting my work, personal life, and health.	**Physical Exam, Stress Management and Complete Medical Evaluation**— Technique designed to alleviate stress and/or increase coping skills	Employee assistant personnel or employee counselor, office medical doctor or nurse, private therapist, stress clinics, caregivers in the workplace, exercise programs

Worksheet adapted from "Care Management Worksheet," *Miles Away and Still Caring*, © 1986, American Association of Retired Persons, pp. 4-5. Reprinted with permission.

Other references published by AARP which your family might find helpful include:

Housing Options for Older Americans
Your Home, Your Choice
Planning Your Retirement Housing
The Right Place at the Right Time
A Handbook About Care in the Home
Healthy Questions
Eating for Your Good Health
The Gadget Book
Information on Medicare and Health Insurance
The Myth of Senility: The Truth About the Brain and Aging
Caregiving, Helping an Aging Loved One
Prepaying Your Funeral

These pamphlets are available from AARP, 601 E Street, NW, Washington, DC 20049. Your local library and social service agencies may have similar publications.

APPENDIX C

NURSING HOME CHECKLIST

You and your family can use this checklist to compare quality of life and care offered by nursing homes you visit prior to placement or to assess the care your parent is receiving once placement has occurred. Because nursing homes may be licensed to offer more than one level of care, always compare similar types of service.

Home A		Home B	
YES	NO	YES	NO

Look at Daily Life

Home A YES	Home A NO	Home B YES	Home B NO	
☐	☐	☐	☐	1. Do residents seem to enjoy being with staff?
☐	☐	☐	☐	2. Are most residents dressed for the season and time of day?
☐	☐	☐	☐	3. Does staff know the residents by name?
☐	☐	☐	☐	4. Does staff respond quickly to resident calls for assistance?
☐	☐	☐	☐	5. Are activities tailored to residents' individual needs and interests?

Home A		Home B		
YES	NO	YES	NO	
☐	☐	☐	☐	6. Are residents involved in a variety of activities?
☐	☐	☐	☐	7. Does the home serve food attractively?
☐	☐	☐	☐	8. Does the home consider personal food likes and dislikes in planning meals?
☐	☐	☐	☐	9. Does the home use care in selecting roommates?
☐	☐	☐	☐	10. Does the nursing home have a resident's council? If it does, does the council influence decisions about resident life?
☐	☐	☐	☐	11. Does the nursing home have a family council? If it does, does the council influence decisions about resident life?
☐	☐	☐	☐	12. Does the facility have contact with community groups, such as pet therapy programs and Scouts?

Look at Care Residents Receive

Home A		Home B		
☐	☐	☐	☐	1. Do various staff and professional experts participate in evaluating each resident's needs and interests?
☐	☐	☐	☐	2. Does the resident (or his or her family) participate in developing the resident's care plan?
☐	☐	☐	☐	3. Does the home offer programs such as physical therapy, occupational therapy, speech and language therapy to restore lost physical functioning?
☐	☐	☐	☐	4. Does the home have any special services that meet your needs, such as special care units for residents with dementia or with respiratory problems?

Home A		Home B		
YES	NO	YES	NO	
☐	☐	☐	☐	5. Does the nursing home have a program to restrict the use of physical restraints?
☐	☐	☐	☐	6. Is a registered nurse available for nursing staff?
☐	☐	☐	☐	7. Does the nursing home have an arrangement with a nearby hospital?

Look at How the Nursing Home Handles Payment

☐	☐	☐	☐	1. Is the facility certified for Medicare?
☐	☐	☐	☐	2. Is the facility certified for Medicaid?
☐	☐	☐	☐	3. Is the resident or the resident's family informed when charges are increasing?

Look at the Environment

☐	☐	☐	☐	1. Is the outside of the nursing home clean and in good repair?
☐	☐	☐	☐	2. Are there outdoor areas accessible for residents to use?
☐	☐	☐	☐	3. Is the inside of the nursing home clean and in good repair?
☐	☐	☐	☐	4. Does the nursing home have handrails in hallways and grab bars in bathrooms?
☐	☐	☐	☐	5. When floors are being cleaned, are warning signs displayed, or are areas blocked off to prevent accidents?
☐	☐	☐	☐	6. Is the nursing home free from unpleasant odors?
☐	☐	☐	☐	7. Are toilets convenient to bedrooms?
☐	☐	☐	☐	8. Do noise levels fit the activities that are going on?

Home A		Home B		
YES	NO	YES	NO	
☐	☐	☐	☐	9. Is it easy for residents in wheelchairs to move around the home?
☐	☐	☐	☐	10. Is the lighting appropriate for what residents are doing?
☐	☐	☐	☐	11. Are there private areas for residents to visit with family, visitors, or physicians?
☐	☐	☐	☐	12. Are residents' bedrooms furnished in a pleasant manner?
☐	☐	☐	☐	13. Do the residents have some personal items in their bedrooms (for example, family pictures, souvenirs, a chair)?
☐	☐	☐	☐	14. Do the residents' rooms have accessible storage areas for residents' personal items?

Other Things to Look For

Home A		Home B		
☐	☐	☐	☐	1. Does the nursing home have a good reputation in the community?
☐	☐	☐	☐	2. Does the nursing home have a list of references?
☐	☐	☐	☐	3. Is the nursing home convenient for family or friends to visit?
☐	☐	☐	☐	4. Does the local ombudsman visit the facility regularly?
☐	☐	☐	☐	5. Is the state health department's annual report posted? What has been done to correct any identified problems?

Adapted from "Nursing Home Checklist," *Guide to Choosing a Nursing Home*, 1993, U.S. Department of Health and Human Services, Health Care Financing Administration, Baltimore, Maryland. (Copies of this publication are available from the HCFA at 7500 Security Boulevard, Baltimore, MD 21244-1850. Write for Publication No. HCFA-02174.)

Issues in Christian Living is a series of six-session study guides that present a Reformed, biblical perspective on life issues that Christians face as they try to live out their Christianity in a society that teaches and models contrary values.

The *Issues in Christian Living* series includes: